Swans in Disguise

You Are Not Fat. You Are Sick.

It is lipedema.

Anna-Theresa Bauer, MD

ISBN-10:1986842010
ISBN-13: **978-1986842013**

To all who suffer from lipedema.

We never know how high we are
Till we are called to rise;
And then, if we are true to plan,
Our statures touch the skies—

The Heroism we recite
Would be a daily thing,
Did not ourselves the Cubits warp
For fear to be a King—

—Emily Dickinson, 1830–1886

Contents

Introduction

Beauty is not in the eye of the beholder anymore. It has become mandatory in our society. Being confronted with various aesthetic surgery issues as a plastic surgery resident, impeccable looks seem to be more important in our society than ever before. To an extent where unhealthy weight ideals are valued and women seem to be put more under pressure to fulfill appearance expectations. Social media is focusing on external beauty and influences our perception through filters everyday creating an illusion that our perfect body is just one diet away. We have become part of a virtual lookbook and our lives are expected to consist of perfect smiles, narrow waists, tiny hips and slim legs.

I must have been fifteen when I came to the conclusion that I was never going to meet any of these expectations again. It was the summer of 2004 when my hips and thighs enlarged dramatically, and I went up three dress sizes in less than two months' time.

My environment told me to be more mindful about my eating habits and to restrict my caloric intake. I exercised every day. I did Pilates and yoga, swam, played tennis, danced, skied in winters, and hiked in summers. I hardly ate, and I remember a time when all I had was a bottle of green tea for breakfast and only one meal per day for many weeks. I basically starved myself. But the size did not change on the lower half of my body, and after some years, I accepted my fate that my legs were constantly growing larger and larger and that I could not wear boots anymore because my calves did not fit into any.

My lower body seemed to swell without any reason. I was a healthy girl but I looked sick and I felt that something was truly wrong with me. The worst thing about that problem were not the irritated looks that people gave me on the streets but the unerring feeling inside me that this was no longer my body. It did somehow not belong to me anymore. I felt like someone had sewn me into a heavy costume of fat tissue without a zipper to unzip and without escape.

Moreover, I developed pain in my lower legs and calves. It was not a bursting pain that sends you immediately to see a doctor, or strong enough to take painkillers, but it was slowly increasing year by year. Worsening throughout the day and especially in summers and lightening in cold times I was not paying too much attention to it most of the time.

I became adapted to it and also to the tingling sensations I felt in my feet after getting up in the morning. I had no explanation for it, I did not feel sick otherwise and I was simply getting used to it. I started to wear compression stockings in my early twenties because I felt kind of a relief of pain and it made my calves look thinner, so I did not give too much thought about it and just incorporated them into my wardrobe.

What stressed me as a teenager and young adult was the fact that I was not able to wear the latest fashion "everybody" was wearing. I just did not fit into the fancy dresses or slim fit jeans that were so trendy. Every time my mother took me shopping, I had grown into a bigger jeans size, so I forced myself onto the next diet. Shopping became a horror event and I ended up with a closet full of black trousers, black dresses, black pullovers and black coats. It was not something I chose because I had a big crush on gothic style but I simply felt better in black stretch trousers than white skinny jeans. Being a slender and joyful child I had turned into a chubby, pale and not so happy teenager who dressed mostly in black. When you are not at ease with your body you want to cover it up and I was feeling comfortable hiding myself in black clothes. Still I swore year-by-year, summer after summer that I would get on a new diet and "next summer" would be better. Sadly, that very good "next summer" never arrived.

It is hilarious how many summers had to pass for me to realize that I had to accept myself the way I was. At some point I simply gave up. I did not see any light or an end of the tunnel.

I had developed a severe eating disorder, which resulted in very unhealthy eating habits varying from binge eating to starvation. Unfortunately, no diet ever showed any long-lasting success, and you might think I had done something wrong, but I read every book on nutrition I could find. At the age of sixteen, I knew the glycemic index and caloric value of every grocery item by heart. I had negative emotions towards food itself and I was far from indulging on any special food. The shame for myself EATING something was so big that I hardly ever ate in public.

Despite a comprehensive education on nutrition that I had received from my parents I could not handle my eating disorder. Eating less did not result in any form of weight loss nor did exercise. So my mind could not connect the dots between caloric intake and weight and slowly surrendered.

Over decades my parents prepared fresh meals daily for us; we grew our own salad, vegetables, and fruit in our garden and they hardly ever took us to fast food restaurants. At that time, my whole family was very skinny, and everybody was doing a lot of sports. The odds of my turning into a "fat" teenager were more than unlikely.

It was not a trauma that happened to me like a car accident, a shooting, or a sudden disease—something that threatens your life or turns it upside down from one moment to another. No, I was hit by something different. I like to compare it to a shadow creeping in or a black veil you do not know how to escape that settles over your life.

It took me almost ten years until I learned what had hit me. Ten years of self doubt and shame. Ten years of fighting a fight you cannot win. My life could have gone a totally different way if somebody had told me earlier that something really was wrong with me. If somebody had told me that I actually suffered from a real disease.

At some point, you are merely existing and not living anymore because the condition keeps making your life so uncomfortable and harder to bear from year to year. It is very hard to describe the subtlety of this disease called lipedema. It is a fat disorder that is progressive and quite unknown to a large part of the population, although a large number of women is affected. And because it is so subtle, it creeps into your life and slowly affects every aspect of it. In a way, it is like a tumor.

First you face the growing thighs and your size enlargement. Then, after you have adjusted to these circumstances, you realize the swelling and pain caused by it. Additionally, you realize the tenderness and easy bruising brought on through inadequate trauma. Besides all of your physical suffering, there is the psychological suffering that continues as you find yourself becoming a person you did not agree to become. You lose control over who you are, and that is scary. No matter how hard you try, no matter how much you exercise or how little you eat the only result is a severe loss of self-confidence. There are many aspects of lipedema that make it an evil disease. It is a disease that affects many women worldwide, yet hardly anybody speaks up about it.

Ten years had passed, and I found myself in a situation that felt like a vacuum. Every single attempt to lose weight and to control my body seemed to be in vain. I found myself trapped in a state of hopelessness. I was far too young, and I did not know what was going on; nobody in my family did. What contributed negatively to my situation of frustration was the lack of understanding I experienced in my family.

They told me that I should stop eating sweets; they advised me to exercise more because with everyone else, the simple rule of caloric intake reduction resulting in weight loss worked—except with me. I felt like an alien among my family and friends. Don't get me wrong—I was never obese. I had a normal BMI at any given time, but my legs and arms enlarged and doubled in size, while my trunk stayed slim.

My legs felt heavy and swollen and cold, even in summer. It was definitely not comparable to obesity in any sense.

There is quite a bit of discussion going on about nutrition and the increase in obesity and diabetes, especially in the younger generations in industrial countries. As a German board-certified specialist doctor in nutrition, I really do agree with the recommendations to eat clean; to cook fresh, local groceries; and to avoid junk food. But why are there still so many women trying to lose weight and, despite years of clean eating, exercising, and going on different diets, starving themselves, growing bigger and bigger?

The ignorance society shows to these ladies is terrifying. I know because I have experienced it. Throughout my life I was an excellent student who lived an active life and I was offered a spot in a medical school in Munich. At the end of medical school, I was twenty-four years old, and without knowing it, I had been sick for almost ten years. The disease was always there in front of everybody's eyes, but nobody had recognized it as a disease. The struggle with weight and jeans and food and guilt had become normal to me. It had begun to define me and become part of my life.

I never imagined I would tell my story to anyone. Indeed, I had the intention of keeping my disease a secret when I learned about it and felt ashamed because of it. There was a moment after suffering over ten years from "being fat" when I realized that it was not my fault. I was neither fat nor undisciplined. I was sick. Finally being diagnosed with a disease called lipedema gave me freedom. It gave me a fighting chance. And step-by-step I learned about the problems the disease can cause, and moreover, I learned that so many women are affected, too, and so few doctors are familiar with it. It was a mixture of happiness, relief, anger, and fear. But the fear was not big enough to keep me from trying to overcome it.

The moment you start realizing it is not your fault, you start fighting it. You start winning. I learned that what had destroyed my self-esteem and confidence over all those years was a fat disorder from which millions of women suffer all over the world. It is called lipedema. "lipos" is Greek, meaning "fat," and "edema" means "swelling/swollen tumor." Finally it all made sense to me. All these years of suffering from the symptoms were related to this disease and yet I had no clue how to deal with it.

I had been privileged enough to become a medical doctor myself and to be assertive enough not to accept the squalid circumstances I had experienced. I sought an explanation and a reason for why my legs looked the way they did.

The first thing I did after being diagnosed in July 2016 was search online for scientific explanations that would help me to understand the disease. But to my disappointment, I could not find them. When I was looking for "lipedema," there were hardly any research results shown. So I started my critical endeavor. I told myself that if I did not start searching for answers to the question of the pathogenesis of my disease, who else would? It seemed like there was very little interest in this disease, and I got very angry. I felt betrayed and left alone by former generations of doctors and scientists who had failed to provide me with sufficient information and understanding about my disease.

Lucky enough I found colleagues in Munich who had specialized in lipedema and diagnosed me with this disease. In the following two years I found the strength to undergo three incredible lipedema surgeries that would change my life more than I had ever expected them to. After fighting the disease and becoming more and more myself, I felt confident enough to talk about it. Moreover, being a plastic surgeon and specialist doctor in nutrition, I started doing experimental research on the disease and asking questions. I could no longer accept the fact that there was no explanation for this disease that everybody just noticed as "fat."

During the last year, I have traveled to many scientific meetings to raise international awareness and gain acknowledgment of this disease—*my* disease.

So besides my own journey as a lipedema patient and a plastic surgeon, I started my career as a lipedema scientist. The motivation could not have been bigger. I felt a sudden connection to all the other women who were out there suffering from this disease and not receiving adequate answers from their doctors. There was a lack of information, and I felt that I had to start contributing to provide answers.

The most shameful comments I heard were those from senior fellow doctors and plastic surgeons. They doubted the mere existence of this disease, but I proved them all wrong. We could show in our recent experiments that lipedema fat cells behave differently than fat cells collected from normal patients who had undergone liposuction for minor cosmetic reasons. I am thankful now because their doubts strongly motivated me to start research on the fat cells. After all, I am grateful for the insults and all the people who doubted me because they ignited my fire to take up a fight against this disease and find its roots.

Moreover I am very grateful to having received research funding from the Lipedema Foundation™ for one of my current science projects analyzing lipedema fat cells on a genetic level, called single cell analysis. The aim of the project is to identify all the genetic information that is within the fat cells from lipedema patients after liposuction and to compare their genome to fat cells from patients who do not suffer from lipedema but have undergone cosmetic liposuction of the same thigh area. We are very curious about the upcoming results.

The tricky thing about lipedema is that there is hardly any common medical knowledge about it, and only a few doctors worldwide have specialized in its treatment. Still, there are so many women and girls who suffer from this disease without knowing it, just like I did for so many years.

Lipedema means constant stress for our bodies, our souls, and our minds. It affects us every single day—sometimes more, sometimes less. But you cannot escape from your body. You want to unzip that heavy fat suit, but you just can't find the zipper. And your daily attempts and efforts to change your diet and to lose that diseased fat make you feel miserable, desperate, and simply lost. This book was written for all of those who need comfort on their journeys struggling with lipedema. It is a navigational light for all of you who feel alone with this disease and so powerless against it. First of all I want you to know that it is not your fault. Lipedema is a real disease.

In the following chapters, you will learn how to recognize lipedema and whether it affects you or anybody in your family. You will subsequently learn what kind of treatment is available at the moment and the state of research that has been done so far. I will give a short introduction into my lipedema diet, which I started after the sick fat had been fully removed and which seems to be working with my "new" metabolism.

Moreover, you will learn how to accept it as your disease, not as your lack of discipline, and you will learn how to deal with it emotionally. It is a revelation to finally embrace your feelings and accept them with all that they comprise.

This book is not a medical textbook, but more of my personal story dedicated to all of you who need comfort in your fight against lipedema when hope seems lost forever. This book is also written for everybody who has a sister, mother, wife, girlfriend or friend suffering from lipedema. I hope that my explanations and emotional insights will help you to understand better how much your support is really needed.

But I also want to share my experiences with you to show you that there is so much strength you can obtain from this struggle and life will be so much better after overcoming lipedema. Know that there is hope and there is a way for us to win. In my opinion lipedema is affecting so many beautiful women and slowly killing their self-esteem and self-love. It is time to change that.

Chapter 1
What Is Lipedema?

When life seems to beat you down, dare to fight back.

-Dr. Steve Maraboli

From a scientific point of view lipedema is a disease mainly affecting women and is characterized by disproportional fat accumulation of the lower extremities and also upper extremities that can result in considerable disability.[1]

In many cases, mothers, grandmothers, sisters, and aunts are affected in a comparable way.[2] The fat pads can extend from the hips to ankles and/or shoulders to wrists and are typically unresponsive to dietary regimes or physical activities.[3] In addition to the aesthetic deformity, women also describe pain in the lower extremities increasing in the course of the day, particularly with tenderness, as well as easy bruising and progressive lymphedema.[4]

Although the disease is well described and an estimated 11 percent of adult women worldwide are affected, it is still often misdiagnosed in a lot of patients.[5] Despite the strong impact of this disease on millions of women's lives, the pathophysiology of this disease is yet unclear. Unlike obesity, the fat cells and swelling associated with lipedema are resistant to change with diet and exercise or bariatric surgery and caloric intake restriction.[5]

One of the typical clinical signs with lipedema is the relative sparing of the feet and hands. As if wearing a bracelet or anklet, the swelling and enlargement of the extremities end at the wrist and ankles, comparable to a cuff.[5]

Although lymphedema might occur as well, especially in higher stages it is also typical that lipedema women can wear normal shoes and do not experience swollen toes and feet.[5]

Moreover, the vessel frailty of lipedema patients has very often been reported, and for most of us, bruising easily when we hit a doorknob or the edge of a table, even though the trauma seems inadequate for that response, has become normal.[5]

As the underlying pathophysiology and "reasons" for this disease are not fully understood there is little I can tell you yet why you suffer from this disease that is affecting so many beautiful women. What we know so far is that there is a growth of the sick fat cells which is called "hypertrophy" and also an increased number of sick fat cells called "hyperplasia".[3]

The reason why we experience swelling in our extremities is not only a result of the growing fat cells but also of the distorted lymphatic system that is becoming leaky and unable to transport the fluid from the tissue.[3]

Lipedema shows 4 major types[3] with 1 to 3 being the most commonly diagnosed. Type 1 affects pelvis, buttocks and hips resulting with an enlargement in these areas disproportional to the rest of the body. Type 2 shows affection from buttocks to knees with nodular tissue and fat pads around the inner thighs and knees. Lumpy fat pads extending from buttocks to ankles affecting the whole lower body characterize type 3. When arms are affected stage 4 is diagnosed.[3]

In my case I was affected with type 4 and I experienced a shifting of types in the course of surgeries. For many years my arms were in a quite steady state regarding size and swelling but suddenly exploded after my first two surgeries when lipedema fat was removed from the lower body.

Another important aspect is the skin texture in lipedema patients as we suffer from nodular fat tissue and lumps that feel like orange peel also known as "cellulitis".[3] I got really concerned when my disease commenced as a teenager and I discovered that not only my thighs showed this texture of the skin but so did my calves.

Due to the lack of information and data on this disease there are only recommendations for treatment options. Conservative treatment includes compression therapy (garments), manual lymphatic drainage and aquatic exercise as well as lifestyle modifications if the lipedema patient is also suffering from obesity. This could be in fact not so easily to distinguish as in higher stages the massive accumulation of fat contributes to weight gain.

The only available treatment to date that has shown long lasting and satisfying results for lipedema patients is surgical liposuction.[5]
After removal of the sick fat pads, patients report an instant lightness in their extremities and a reduction of cellulitis, swelling, pain, and bruising as well as metabolic improvements.[2]

Moreover many patients report an aesthetic improvement and an overall improvement in life quality.[2] Regarding my own experiences after lipedema surgery I will elaborate on that in the following chapters.

Results from a recent study showed so far that lipedema did not come back after follow-ups of 85 patients eight years after lipedema surgery.[6]

In another study, a total of 112 lipedema patients were reviewed approximately three years after lipedema surgery and showed a distinct improvement of shape and body proportions as well as a marked improvement or complete disappearance of spontaneous pain or sensitivity to pressure, bruising, and restriction of movement.[7-10] Another fact about lipedema is that a positive family history has been reported in many cases, pointing out a genetic background of the disease not fully discovered yet.

A study from 2010 showed that within six families affecting more than three generations with lipedema a genetic hereditary pattern was found.[11]

I believe that lipedema has existed over the decades, for a very long time. I remember my grandmother always wearing long skirts and complaining about pain in her legs, especially after long walks. My grandfather literally carried her on Sunday afternoon walks when her legs hurt so much that she could not go on. She was misdiagnosed with venous insufficiency and got her veins stripped three times. Nobody knew that this disease even existed fifty years ago. When I told my father about my lipedema problem, he was very comforting and said, "Yes, I believe you. I remember that your grandmother's legs looked the same as yours." He was one of the few people I did not have to convince that my condition being a disease. So I believe a lot of grandmothers and mothers were suffering for many years from this disease that today we call lipedema, but due to a lack of medical knowledge, they were never diagnosed or their complaints were completely misinterpreted and therefore misdiagnosed. Nowadays, generations of women have access to various sources of medical information, and I will fight along with other people to make lipedema more commonly known. Informing doctors, as well as patients, about lipedema is important because more and more women will be alerted by their symptoms and they cannot find medical help if their doctors are not educated in a proper manner. It will be a long time until medical textbooks will include lipedema—or maybe a few already have—but I am of the opinion that it is worth the challenge.

Chapter 2

Are You One of Us?

*A group of thoughtful people could change the world.
Indeed, it's the only thing that ever has.*

- Margaret Mead

So what about you? Can you relate to the symptoms I described in the previous chapter? Do you also suffer from "tree trunk" legs and feel like your body is not your "true body"? Does the swelling and pain gets worse throughout the day, especially in your legs? Do you suffer from tenderness and easy bruising when you hit the doorknob with your arm or somebody pulls you slightly?

Do you sometimes find your legs covered with black and blue marks (hematoma) and you cannot remember where they came from? Have you tried every fancy diet in the world, and still your efforts to lose weight in the particular areas of your body are fruitless? Do you feel ashamed of yourself when you look in the mirror and often hear comments from friends and family that you are probably just not trying hard enough?

First of all, and most importantly, I know exactly how you feel. I have been there for many years, and I know the feeling: Unsure whether it is just my lack of discipline or destiny is playing a bad joke on me. Wondering why it is not getting better over time but worse and worse. Gaining more and more weight, especially on my legs and hips. Slowly but continuously—that's what we call "progressive" in medicine. You cannot stop it. You cannot prevent it from coming. You can only accept it.

The worst thing about lipedema was not the pain, the swelling, or the looks other people gave me on the streets in summer. The worst thing was the complete loss of control over my own body. As you experience failure after failure when intending to lose weight, you become more and more fatalistic, and you feel powerless. This feeling can affect every aspect of your life.

In addition to my own experiences I want to share some facts with you. We conducted the biggest lipedema online survey in Europe in 2017, asking questions of 1,193 female patients who had been diagnosed with lipedema and not been operated on thus far. Many patients felt annoyed and angry because they did not receive any financial aid and moreover because they had been suffering for so many years and nobody had diagnosed them earlier. This is a huge problem as lipedema surgeries cost thousands of dollars and insurance companies do not cover the costs usually.

The average lipedema patients were female and thirty-eight years old. They reported that their diseases had first manifested at the average age of sixteen. It took them a mean of fifteen years to get diagnosed by a board-certified doctor and lipedema specialist. In 99 percent of all cases thighs were the region affected and, in 86 percent, calves. In 82 percent of all cases, upper arms were affected and, in 35 percent, forearms. Belly fat was affected in 43 percent of cases, and 15 percent of patients reported an affection of the back (region of bra closures). The median weight of participants was one hundred kilograms with a standard deviation of twenty-five kilograms. We were also very interested in comorbidities and asked about a variety of common diseases or allergies. A total of 42.4 percent of lipedema women stated they were affected by allergies, for example. This may seem a lot, but in fact it is a normal percentage compared to the average prevalence of allergic diseases of German average women thirty to thirty-nine years old with a percentage of 42.2.[12]

Another comorbidity questioned was polycystic ovary syndrome, a complex gynecological disease that affects ovaries and can cause infertility. As it is sometimes referred to as the "metabolic syndrome of the ovaries," we were curious about the coincidence, but only 4.7 percent stated they were diagnosed with this disease. So from that we can draw the conclusion that lipedema fat is not only resistant to diets and exercise but also the average lipedema patient is kind of a healthy person and for the most part not suffering from any metabolic diseases.

Thirty-three percent of patients reported suffering from depression, and 35 percent suffered from hypothyroidism. This is clearly over the average, which is about 2 to 4 percent of the normal population.[13]

I think depression is an important topic regarding lipedema as with the disease there comes a feeling of desperation and isolation. I will elaborate on this subject in one of the following chapters also providing tips how to deal with feelings of hopelessness and anxiety.

Regarding the hypothyroidism there is an interesting link between hypothyroidism which means a distorted function of the thyroid glands producing not enough hormones to provide essential body functions.[13] What we see in severe cases of hypothyroidism is also called "myxedema" and is seen also in the pretibial region, the front side of the calves.[13] Now as one of the alarm signs in lipedema described in the diagnostic manual resembles pretibial myxedema extraordinarily.

In our survey results showed no significant elevation of metabolic diseases in the comorbidities among lipedema patients; only 2 percent suffered from diabetes mellitus type II, and 0.5 percent stated they suffered from diabetes type I. Only 7 percent reported elevated levels of cholesterol. These results are interesting in my opinion, as lipedema fat might be detached from the body's metabolism and therefore not clinically correlating with abnormal levels of glucose, which would result in a higher prevalence of diabetes or elevated levels of cholesterol. So conclusively lipedema women seem to be quite healthy overall and that is also what I can agree with.

I have seen several other lipedema patients presenting in higher stages. They had already developed lip-lymphedema and lip sclerosis, and they were desperate, but on the other hand, they were also very glad to be finally taken serious by doctors who did not tell them to lose weight and start exercising. However, I strongly recommend treating lipedema at an early stage because the outcome can be amazing. I never before could have imagined the relief I experienced after surgery.

Another aspect of "lipedema women" I find important to mention here is that many of my lipedema patients and fellow sufferers are extremely kind-hearted and nice people. You might think that is by chance, but I think lipedema has really prevented us from becoming superficial and nasty. We cannot rely on our looks matching the typical beauty ideals. That's maybe why we have to excel in other qualifications and develop our characters in order to make up what we lack in superficial beauty idealism.

Whoever thinks that a girl with lipedema will end up unhappy and lonely is on the other hand completely wrong. I did not collect any data on this topic, but that is just my opinion from what I experienced and witnessed. I am very grateful that a lot of men still look beyond dress sizes and recognize the beauty they find in women with lipedema because we are beautiful swans hidden underneath a few layers of sick fat. Be grateful for those who see you like this and do not try to change you because they think you are not motivated enough to exercise more or eat less because they want you to fit into a certain dress size. Be thankful for them. They will be happy for you when you finally shed your diseased fat that does not really belong to you. Nobody will ever understand. Don't expect it from anybody who does not suffer from lipedema. Just be grateful for those who accept, support, and love you.

So I had to find other positive traits of my personality to keep up a minimum of self-esteem to achieve all of my daily goals, and I am thankful for the people who always loved and accepted me the way I was no matter how I looked. I think a lot of lipedema women are superwomen without acknowledging it. Think about it for a moment. Millions of women are respected members of our society, build families, have amazing careers, live their lives to the fullest, and try to do everything as well as or even better than other women despite their burden of lipedema. Please do not confuse lipedema with obesity. Being overweighed is not a nice situation for your body, but does not have to be a burden. Moreover patients do not suffer from this certain "lipedema pain" and all the other symptoms lipedema brings with it. Lipedema patients know exactly what I mean. I was never obese, I never had any other disease before in my life and I was a high performer in a stable social environment. It is easier for many people to believe that you are just lazy and tired than to acknowledge the fact that there is a "new" disease that nobody has heard about before. That's why it is so important to talk about lipedema and to get engaged in the discussion.

To bring you closer to the understanding of what lipedema feels like, I want you to join me on this imaginative journey: Imagine a hot, sunny summer day when you get up in the morning and know it is going to be too warm to wear long trousers. With lipedema legs, that day is a nightmare.

Summer after summer, I counted the days until autumn approached and cooler temperatures settled in. My favorite time of the year was autumn because you still had the sun and sixty-degree Fahrenheit weather (around fifteen degrees Celsius). I was so glad when every summer was over; no one can imagine. Most of the time in summer, I stayed inside my house with the shutters closed and the air-conditioning on. Working in the clinic without air-conditioning was not so easy, but I wore compression stockings under my scrubs to reduce the swelling, which seemed ridiculous to anyone else who did not suffer from lipedema. It was a life I got very used to. I was so limited in my choices, and in summertime I did not live; I merely existed. I hoped for rainy, cool summers when others were all about holidays and sunshine.

Going swimming was impossible. In the early days of lipedema I still had enough self-confidence to push myself into a bathing suit and to the beach. But people started to stare at my swollen ankles and I felt so shameful. At some point I just stopped wearing skirts or swimwear.

My abstinence from the sun got so severe that I developed a sun allergy, first presenting during a week on beach vacation in 2012 when I was first exposed to sunlight after a couple of summers without it. Moreover, I developed a lack of vitamin D, which is crucial for many important physiological functions. Not only had lipedema isolated me from the normal people who went to the beach in summers and were able to wear skirts and sleeveless shirts, but it also started to affect my health on a deeper level.

Lipedema isolates you and is like a slowly creeping death for your social life. I had to find excuses for why I was not "in the mood" to go swimming or on holidays or why I wanted to go straight home from work to the cool, dark house. Every evening, I found myself staying at home with my legs elevated, reading, watching a movie, or working. I believe most of you have had similar experiences.

Besides the swelling, I started realizing an aching in my joints when I walked more than one hour. I felt like an old lady. I was twenty-five years old and had the physique of an eighty-five-year-old woman. I knew something was going in the wrong direction here. I knew I should be running every day or enjoying any kind of sportive hobby to relax and just have fun. Instead, I was aching from day to day, and all I could do was go to work and come back home to lie down. As a surgical resident, that is what you usually do anyway, but compared to other residents, I was not living my life. I was enduring. I was waiting for my life to become better someday.

For many years I was not sure why felt the way I did and I simply could not find explanations for my symptoms because nobody had recognized them as part of a complex disease called lipedema.

In the following chapter you will learn how to recognize lipedema, and I will explain the symptoms more detailed and also from my personal point of view.

Chapter 3

How to Recognize It

*We cannot change what we are not aware of, and once
we are aware, we cannot help but change.*

—Sheryl Sandberg

I hereby state that lipedema is probably one of the
most misdiagnosed and undiagnosed diseases in the
world. It is a disease that can isolate people and drive
them further away from their true personalities. It is a
real tragedy that doctors often do not look further for
the reason women complain about swollen extremities,
suffer from constant weight gain especially in the
extremities, are frustrated with trying to lose weight,
and experience a tendency to bruise easily.

There is a saying in medical school: "When you hear
hoof beats, think of horses, not zebras." Even though
most doctors see a lot of patients suffering from
obesity, they should never forget that lipedema women

are like zebras. They exist and need to be recognized and correctly diagnosed.

The German Society of Phlebology has found consensus in 2017 once again that the diagnosis of lipedema should be made upon patient history and clinical findings.[14]

But how can a disease be correctly diagnosed when a lot of doctors still don't know about the symptoms? And how, as a lipedema patient, can you prove that you are actually sick and not fat if nobody believes you? One of the biggest challenges for future studies is to provide a reliable and objective test (e.g., genetic test) for lipedema.

One of the biggest problems I recognized during my journey was the ignorance of many doctors, and it was not so easy to find a doctor who had the experience to diagnose lipedema. In Germany, we are blessed to have a lot of specialized board-certified doctors. In Europe, we excel in the medical field by setting certain standards in patient care and pushing the edge in science. At least that was what I thought before I tried to find a doctor who could tell me what was wrong with my legs and arms. I remember sitting on a gynecologist's chair with my legs exposed to the old doctor whom I really respected for his years of medical experience. When he saw my swollen legs and puffy knees, he sighed and said, "Oh, dear, your legs look exactly like those my daughter has. She is a doctor, too, but there is nothing you can do about it. Just accept it." I broke out in tears. It hurt so much, and I could not cope with that feeling for a very long time. One of the worst feelings humans can experience is hopelessness, I guess, and I felt so hopeless back then. I'm sure many of you know what I mean.

For years, I did not accept my legs. I tried to work out regularly and even hired a personal trainer. Going to the gym always seemed like a threat to me. In a way it stole my energy instead of enhancing my energy. I could never understand why people liked to work out and had fun exercising. For me the real torture started when I hit the gym and had to face all these mirrors around me reflecting my disproportionate body. Moreover I had to wear compression stockings to prevent heavy legs and swelling in my calves after exercise. It was not until after my first lipedema surgery that I started to have fun going to the gym and felt like a normal person with normal calves and ankles. This was a one-of-a-kind experience.

After the disease got worse in 2016, I started another attempt to find a doctor who could tell me what was wrong with my legs. As a plastic surgeon, I have to stand for hours, and despite wearing compression stockings every day, my legs hurt more and more in the evenings. I could not help it or accept it any longer. I had to go find a specialist doctor. In my case, it was even more difficult to overcome the shame of suddenly being a patient, standing on the other side.

As a doctor, you don't get to be the patient. You are not allowed to whine or complain or take days off when you are suffering a cold or whatever. You just don't get to be sick. You don't have the right to be. You need to behave like a kind of superhuman. But lipedema does not care about your profession, whether you are a doctor or an IT specialist or a full-time mother. It can also affect women of any age.

So my next appointment was in the summer of 2016. It was with a female phlebologist, and it was one of the most horrible experience I'd had in a very long time. The doctor was about fifty years old; she said she was a marathon runner, and worst of all, she had zero knowledge about lipedema or compassion for my suffering. She examined my veins and told me that my veins worked perfectly fine but I just should stop eating so much chocolate cream and start working out on a daily basis. She suggested running. She said she did not believe in lipedema and that most of the problems were related to a dietary issue. If somebody had slapped me in the face, it would have been easier to handle and less painful for me than her suggestions. But I did not give up and luckily found another phlebologist, who reassured me that my veins were operating just fine but that I clearly suffered from lipedema.

Although lipedema is not a rare condition lipedema is often misdiagnosed as lymphedema or obesity.[14]
A lot of doctors raise the specter of doubt when it comes to lipedema because they claim you can't differentiate between an obese woman and a woman suffering from lipedema. Well, I can understand them; if they have not seen many lipedema patients in their careers so far, it can be quite tricky.

Part of my endeavor is to raise awareness in the medical and scientific community, and I am not alone in this. I know lipedema specialists who also organize meetings and constantly try to elaborate better standards in order to make it easier for other doctors to diagnose lipedema correctly. But those of you who have experienced every symptom of this disease on your own bodies might just be the best lipedema experts ever.

Here are some diagnostic criteria I will explain to you. Just as I experienced them firsthand, maybe you can also check a lot of them on your list:

1) One of the primary indicators for lipedema is a disproportion of your small waist, large buttocks, and trunk-shaped legs. In our study of twelve hundred patients, there was a significant difference between the lower body and the upper body, measuring three dress sizes in average. The waist-to-hip ratio is usually lower than 0.7. It is furthermore characterized by localized adiposity with an increase of subcutaneous fat tissue.[14] With progression of the disease, the belly can also turn into an affected area. That is why lipedema patients are mostly not obese in the early stages. Their trunks show their real size, while extremities are out of the range. There is a significant discrepancy between the upper body (trunk) and the lower body such as thighs

and calves; in higher stages, the upper arms
and forearms can also be affected. Lipedema
can solely affect forearms, upper arms, or both.
There is a significant border between my wrists
and forearms. In my case, the lower extremities
were affected first, and after removal of the
diseased fat, the affected areas of the upper
arms and forearms got even worse. It was like
my body realized that it could not store any
sick fat in the legs once it was gone.

2) The typical swelling ("edema") occurs mainly
in the extremities, sparing the hands and feet.[5]
The most common signs I always look for in
patients are their knees and ankles. I could not
see my anklebones anymore, and my kneecap
(patella) was hidden under a bunch of nodular
fat tissue. If your hands and feet are affected,
too, it might not be lipedema but lymphedema.
However, please do yourself a favor and have
your veins, heart, and renal function examined.
Peripheral swelling (edema) can also result

from pathology of one of these organs. If your veins are not showing any signs of insufficiency and your other organs are working fine as well, your swelling will most probably derive from lipedema if you suffer from other symptoms, too. An important sign is Stemmer's sign: it is a positive sign for lymphedema but negative for lipedema. To perform it you try to pinch and lift a skinfold at the base of the second toe. If you can pinch and lift the skin, Stemmer's sign is negative. If you can't the sign is positive.[5]

3) Skin surface and skin elasticity is an important issue, too. The skin texture is granular to palpation with nodular fat lumps increasing with time.[3] When correctly performed ultrasound can distinguish between normal fat tissue and lipedema fat tissue showing enlarged chambers of fat (septa). Healthy fat tissue follows pressure easily compared to lipedema fat, which is so swollen due to edema.

Moreover the lipedema skin loses its elasticity and fat accumulates in nodules and little pockets especially over the joints.

4) Moreover lipedema women appear also to suffer from teleangiectasia above average.[5] That's what we call the little spider veins that are not pathognomonic for lipedema and they have no pathological influence.

5) One of the most important diagnostic findings is of course pain.[1] Pain can vary from 1-10 VAS (ten maximum) and many lipedema women describe it as a pain near 7-8 VAS. I have to mention that pain is a crucial parameter in my opinion but there have been also cases described who did not suffer from any pain. In my case the pain was around VAS 2-3.

6) Another problem is the fragility of vessels and the resulting easy bruising after inadequate trauma. The reason for this vessel fragility is

not clear yet. Scientists from Hungary found in 2012 that lipedema is associated with increased aortic stiffness, and there might exist a microangiopathy, a kind of defect and instability of the small vessel membrane.[16] However, what it causes is what annoys us in the form of hematoma and easy bruising when hitting a doorknob or a chair.

7) There is kind of a common ground in the lipedema community that the disease starts with puberty or times of hormonal change such as pregnancy, hormone therapy (also getting on the pill), and menopause.[1] We have not yet identified the genes that are affected, and there might be a trigger for the disease deriving from hormonal imbalances, but almost 50 percent of our twelve hundred lipedema patients stated in the survey that their disease started at the beginning of puberty. In my case, I can relate to that experience, as my lipedema started when I was fifteen years old. I also experienced

a significant aggravation of lipedema fat pads when I got on the pill and a relief when I stopped the intake. You might also experience aggravation when getting pregnant or after menopause.

8) Lipedema fat is resistant to radical dieting and fasting. Forty percent of our surveyed German patients stated they were following a special diet. Diets stated were low carb, gluten free, ketogenic diet, HCG, Weight Watchers, and others. Forty-five percent of the surveyed women of the British study in 2014 reported suffering from eating disorders.[17] There is no scientific evidence that any of these dietary regimes ever showed a significant improvement in lipedema patients, and more clinical data is needed. Scientists showed in 2009 that lipedema fat cells seem to be microscopically surrounded by an increase of inflammatory cells.[15]

9) What is important to mention is that with lipedema patients often witness a kind of lipedema fatigue, as an easy tiring of physical activities and a progressive deterioration of mobility. Also cold sensations can be noticed. My thighs always felt cooler than the trunk.

Now that you know more about the disease from what has been elaborated so far and how I experienced them it is time for us to take a look at how you can handle it. Never doubt that you can get out of this body that does not feel like it is yours—because you can, and by the end of reading this book, you will know how to manage it.

Chapter 4

Is Anybody Out There?

To be alone is to be different, to be different is to be alone.

\- Suzanne Gordon

Eighty-one percent of our almost twelve hundred lipedema patients felt misunderstood for their disease in their environment. This is something we have to change. I am very grateful that there is a lipedema movement getting bigger, raising awareness in society for this disease. In Connecticut, a nongovernmental private family organization called the Lipedema Foundation™ was established in 2015; the foundation is a strong financial and scientific supporter of lipidema scientists all over the world and has been a powerful advocate for lipedema women since 2013 and for increased awareness of the disease, especially in the United States.

In recent years, there has luckily been the rise of a new lipedema movement. A British study in 2014 asked 250 lipedema women to complete a seventy-four-question survey.[17] They found that 86 percent of the surveyed lipedema patients suffered from low self-esteem; 60 percent reported restricted social lives and feelings of hopelessness. This is something I really shared. And the reason I think it is important to mention that here is that if you suffer from that, too, you should know it is normal.

It is a symptom of your disease in my opinion. It took me a very long time to acknowledge this and accept it for myself.

If you are not familiar with the disease because nobody else in your family has been suffering from it so far, you feel lost, alone, and hopeless, just like I did. My grandmother died when I was five years old. I did not get the chance to talk to her about her legs or lipedema when I came into puberty experiencing the symptoms for the first time. My social life got so restricted I could not go out in the evening to dance or wear high heels. My legs were extremely swollen, they hurt, and I sensed a tingling sensation in the morning sometimes when I had night shifts and was up on my feet all night. I was feeling more and more isolated, and my friends did not know why I refused many of their evening invitations.

In the British lipedema study, 50 percent reported restrictions in their sex lives, and in our German survey, it was 69 percent. Imagine how many problems in romantic relationships could vanish if women did not suffer from their constant pain, swollen legs, and low self-confidence and simply got rid of their sick lipedema fat.

Seventy percent of the lipedema women from our German survey stated that they had serious problems due to pain in their legs when walking for longer than one hour. Compression garments are crucial for lipedema women when exercising or walking long distances in order to reduce and prevent swelling. Survey respondents stated a mean time of eleven hours per day for their time of compression. I think many non-lipedema women cannot imagine a life wearing compression almost the entire day, but compression stockings became normal to my wardrobe.

Many times when I was preparing for competitions, job interviews, or congresses, I had to go shopping, and I jealously glimpsed the knee-length skirts and sleeveless dresses. I always went for wide dark blue or black trousers and long-sleeved blouses. I cannot say I did not look decent, but I was so limited in my choices of what to wear that it broke my heart every time such an event approached. Ninety-five percent of lipedema sufferers in the British poll reported that they had difficulties buying clothes. If you feel the same way, welcome to our circle of understanding. Separate from people who are reluctant to understand your disease or not willing to support you. Such people simply keep you from moving forward and healing. No matter how much it hurts, keep them out and trust in yourself.

There will be supporters along the way. I am one of them.

Talking about support—use the power of social media. Get in touch with other lipedema women. Facebook groups provide lipedema patients space for communication and exchange of thoughts, photos, and problems. Never underestimate the power of a community. It is psychological support in times when nobody in the world seems to understand you and society seems reluctant to understand. I met a fellow patient in the hospital on the day I had my first liposuction done. She was a very kind and intelligent lady in her forties, and after we introduced ourselves, lying there in our beds after these very exhausting surgeries, we instantly became friends. The same fate often ties bonds that we could not have expected before. So get connected. You are not alone.

In fact dealing with this disease on a more conscious level will make you stronger. Never doubt that this is not for you. As I mentioned before self-doubt and a lack of self-esteem are the major problems that come with lipedema. So what can you do about it? Self-trust can be described as the reliance on your own personality, ability, strength and truth. The problem is, with lipedema most of us have spent many years listening to other people believing them that we are just "too lazy" or not "consequent enough" to push through our daily exercise or to keep track on our diet. We have been conditioned to the idea that we are doing something wrong and we do not know what is best for ourselves. Instead we believe people who we think know more about us and we try to live accordingly to what they think is "true".

We allow ourselves to be who we are told that we are: Lazy, fat, not beautiful, and not enough. We get so caught up in this endless struggle for approval and reaching for recognition that the result is we simply lose trust in our inner voice and ourselves. The result of believing other's opinion more than what we feel is torture. I believe that this is one of the most painful states of mind. This kind of self-distrust creates suffering because the root of the problem is that we do not trust ourselves anymore. This goes hand in hand with a lack of self-confidence.

When people use the word confidence, they often mean the ability to depend on yourself. If you don't have self-confidence, you won't feel able to rely on yourself. This means you do not trust yourself because your body feels out of control and therefore you easily let others take control over you with their opinion. This leads further to a lack of self worth and is an issue of invalidating yourself. In other words we are not able to see our own value anymore. So in a way blaming other people for not taking you and your struggle with lipedema serious is in the end a struggle with yourself.

But how can you stop this vicious circle? My advice is to listen to your feelings and not to suppress the negative emotions any longer. Instead – embrace them. I know the fear and the anxiety of going to public places. I know the disgust you feel when you look in the mirror at your oversized disproportionate body.

I know how deep these emotions cut into your soul. Our feelings mirror us. Many people have forgotten their most accurate sense of their emotions and sensations.

So it has become natural to suppress feelings, especially negative ones. And with lipedema there comes a whole bunch of negative feelings. But the beautiful truth is that emotions are also the compass to our lives and our true destiny. Your duty is to feel and allow your emotions to tell you their message.

They are all the guidance we need. It is only when we ignore them for a long time that we become somehow convinced that they have failed us. So for example in the case of lipedema we have lost our self trust and therefore self worth and we end up depending on how other people define us which leads into a feeling of powerlessness and struggle. So how can we change that?

In the following chapter, you will learn what helped me deal with the diagnosis and what is important to learn for accepting your situation and allowing your feelings in order to transform yourself.

Chapter 5

How to Deal with the Disease

When fear disappears, the foundation of disease is gone.

- Mary Baker Eddy

Once you have been diagnosed, one of the most important things to learn is that no matter how bad it has been, there is finally light at the end of the tunnel. Years of denial, self-doubt and blame are finally over. No matter how many emotional scars you are carrying already, you have proven to be a strong woman because you put up a fight with yourself every day. Think about it in a new way: you are eligible to suffer from lipedema because you are strong enough to take it.

You are special in a way that only few are and are blessed to get a chance to overcome this disease and, thus, every shadow of self-consciousness, doubt, and self-hatred. It is time to heal and to take action to fight this disease. You can turn your weakness into your superpower. This is what I like to call transformation and I will show you how to achieve that.

Before I had been diagnosed I found myself in an alternating state of hopelessness and anger. Hopelessness is one of the cruelest feelings one can experience. Congratulations to all of the lipedema ladies who feel the same – we hit the jackpot of worst emotions. Feeling hopeless can lead people into depression and anxiety disorders and in rare cases even into suicide. But why is it so powerful that we hardly can handle or escape? Because it is a feeling that tells you unconsciously that you will suffer forever.

This causes your mind to think this is the end and there will be only pain and suffering also in the future. This feeling of hopelessness is often deeply rooted in our early days with lipedema when we made our first negative experiences and got into the vicious circle of self doubt and low self worth leading to a loss of hope. Be assured – anyone who has experienced lipedema struggles with hopelessness from time to time or even constantly. It is important for you to know that nothing is wrong with you if you feel that way. It merely reflects the condition you are in and these thoughts you are thinking are a simple result of it. So when you are feeling hopeless you have already entered the attitude "whatever I try nothing ever works". But what can you do about it?

You can either distract yourself actively by creating a new mindset and focusing on something really important like an activity you are working on. This could be organizing a children's birthday party or planning any other social event that really needs your attention and gets you short time off the hook of hopelessness. For me it has always been and still is my work as a doctor.

Another very helpful exercise you can practice is to take one step back and distance from your emotions. You need to dis-identify with your thoughts and step into an observational state of mind. This has helped me several times when I felt like drowning in despair. I closed my eyes and took a deep breath an imagined myself from an outside perspective. How do I look like to someone else outside my body? Is my situation really that hopeless? I then focused and tried to count my blessings like: I am a healthy young intelligent female with a great job and a great family and amazing friends… so on. Sometimes you just need to change your perspective and your mind changes. It can be incredibly effective in a moment of a negative spiral of thoughts. Every time you feel that hopelessness creeping in try to focus on counting your blessings.

Another exercise that helped me tremendously when I found myself crying in front of a mirror because of my lipedema legs was to stop that momentum of hopelessness and forced myself to smile at myself. With all due respect to the human brain but it can be tricked. When you are feeling such negative emotions that you cannot think of anything positive about yourself, start to smile and the world will change.

The moment your brain realizes it gets a positive impression and feedback you will realize some profound change. To put it short notice: You have to end this fight with yourself.

Because no matter how cursed your body seems and how bad your situation is, the more you resist it the longer you will have to fight against yourself.

Acceptance is the first step toward living a normal life despite lipedema. It is much easier to shame us for being lazy with exercise, indulging our sweet tooth too often, or finding other excuses than to accept it. I want you to stop this shaming because it is not true. It is not your fault; it never has been and never will be. It is a genetically preconditioned disease that affects so many of us. Society has not acknowledged it yet, but times are changing with every one of us.

Feeling lost and unsure is part of your struggle. Don't avoid it. Instead, see what those feelings are showing you and use them. Even if you feel a hundred times like you are drowning in despair because of this disease, believe me, you won't. You will be just fine. One of the most important things you have to learn is how to stop caring what other people think about you.

Throughout the time as a lipedema patient you will receive judgment from other people, whether you like it or not. I used to have a very thin skin. Like a bullet, every disapproving word or action directed at me by others hit me straight to my core. I felt more than affected by it. I would have loved to be more unaffected by other people's opinions and actions, but I was not. If you're that kind of person, too, it is not a conscious choice to not be hurt by something someone says. And thinking that it is a conscious choice, will merely make you feel guilty about feeling bad. In a way we have conditioned our behavior over the past years. We were rewarded for good behavior with treats, and punished for bad behavior. For some of us, there were big consequences when the people in our early lives disapproved of us.

Probably our boundaries were violated. We got either hurt by incoming boundary violation, such as insults or shaming comments resulting in issues with caring what other people think. The message we learned was that we did not deserve love of others if we were not pleasing them. This is a big issue when we remember that love is mandatory for our personal growth and happiness, especially when we were dependent on others like in our childhood. To our minds, disapproval back then meant failure. When we grow up, it doesn't change. Disapproval still means failure.

A lot of people will tell you to "stop taking it so personally," which is an assault that minimizes how you feel. But why do we take things personally? Because back when we were children, when we did something wrong, we were told that we failed. When we did something that our parents disapproved of, our parents disapproved of us as people, not just the action that upset them. We learned it really was personal. Doing something wrong made us consecutively bad people. Doing something bad made us bad. So now, we have serious issues with rejection and disapproval because our self-esteem was and still is essentially dependent on approval.

You are not going to heal your wounds, learn how to validate yourself and stop being negatively affected by what other people think with one autosuggestion technique or with a magic pill. This is a healing process which gets better and better every day. Everything begins with the knowledge that it is okay to feel hurt because of what someone has said or done. You can't control what others do, what they say or think. But you can consciously choose how to treat yourself and what to do with yourself when you have been hurt by someone. And if you chose to approach that task differently, being wounded by others can open the perfect opportunity to healing and self-integration. And once we seize this opportunity, we will not have the same painful reaction to the judgments of others.

After this journey, you will definitely not be the same person you were when you started the adventure. Once you enter on this road, you will be in a constant process of change. You will realize that people around you will lose their importance. People who kept your self-esteem low will lose their power over you and your self-worth. They will vanish. You will become more and more yourself while abandoning your old body with every layer of sick fat. At the end of this chapter of your life, you can turn the page and breathe. You will feel like yourself again, like you have never imagined before. The physical pain that has become so overwhelmingly emotional will decrease, and you will be able to live a life without constant self-doubts, self-hatred, and pain. If this sounds unreal to you, it is the best indication to continue reading and get into the process.

Resistance has been part of your history as a lipedema woman for long enough. Try to avoid resistance in order to accept yourself. This may sound very easy, but in fact, it is one of the hardest things to learn, and it took me over one year of ups and downs to finally come to the point of full acceptance for myself and my body. Some of you might have experienced incredible torture of your self-confidence and obstacles in your professional lives because of lipedema-associated problems.

There is a very good practice of gaining self-love I once read about and I want to share it with you in order to come to acceptance and self-approval. It may sound difficult to you, but in fact, it can really help. It is a really simple procedure. All you need is a glass full of water or your favorite tea. Focus on the fluid inside the glass for a few moments and imagine inside this glass is a special fluid that contains pure love for yourself.

When you have focused enough, you are ready to drink, and you should swallow the fluid very slowly. With every sip, you should focus on the love running down inside your body, filling you with love. Sip at least ten times and try to feel yourself better with every sip. When I first heard about this thing, I laughed very hard and thought that would be great if the mind could be "tricked" like this—drinking water and feeling more beloved. But then I tried it and after a few times, I really felt a difference. Drinking water can serve as not only a way to stay hydrated, but also a method to help you focus on and create a deeper connection with yourself.

This is only one example of many on this practice of self-love and acceptance. But if you want to fully come to terms with the diagnosis, it is inevitable and necessary to accept yourself and start loving yourself.

Deep down we might have felt unworthy to be loved because of our lipedema legs because we thought we were flawed. For a long time this was not obvious to me and I had developed patterns of behavior that I never had given a second thought of. For instance I had become more and more altruistic to an unhealthy extent. When I went out for dinner or lunch with my girls I always wanted to take the bill and pay for all of us because I felt so grateful they had spent time with me that in a way I thought I would owe them now at least to pay for the dinner.

They never understood and laughed and of course shared the bills many times. I could not believe that somebody actually would like to spend time with me and that was ridiculous. It took me a very long time to feel comfortable to be invited.

But it is true - you have to love yourself first before you can accept the love of others. Throughout my life I had been a giver in relationships. I always gave more than I received. All I longed for was to be appreciated and to be likeable. It took me a long time to discover that lipedema had had such a deep impact on my behavior.

So what can you learn from that? If you recognize similar patterns of behavior or feelings within you, please notice that you are not alone and it is most probably because of lipedema. You need to step outside your body one more time and start re-building your vision of yourself. This will give you more and more self-esteem. It will empower you to look beyond your lipedema legs and whenever you speak badly of yourself – stop. Ponder your words and realize that it is "lipedema" talking. You are strong and brave and try to regain power over your thoughts.

In my opinion your thoughts are your reflection of your beliefs and they shape your behavior. I made the mistake for too many years to speak or think badly of myself because I thought I was "flawed" due to lipedema.

I wish for every one of you who shares that problem that she will step up with me and stop that negative vibes. Sometimes we are ourselves worst enemies and our biggest critics.

There was a time when I tried to convince myself that I could handle lipedema without undergoing surgery. I told myself over and over again that I was smart enough and disciplined enough to follow any diet and do any kind of exercise that would shrink my lipedema fat pads. But I was wrong. Round after round my confidence was smashed when I discovered after another few weeks that in fact nothing had changed or it had even gotten worse. There was that point of maximum desperation that I needed to stop negotiating with myself and accept that only surgical removal of the fat via liposuction could be the game changer.

Maybe in earlier stages it can be possible to handle lipedema without surgery. In my case I had suffered from it for 10 years and it had reached such an extent that the disease had manifested and conservative therapy did not have any impact on me anymore. I have read about cases where women managed to contain lipedema solely with special forms of nutrition and compression garments.

I believe there is not simply one problem about lipedema. There are many. And it can be really challenging to deal with all of them at the same time.

I like to compare it to an onion. When you peel it, starting from the outside, there is society, who only sees your oversize legs or arms or body in general. Some people may act judgmental; others simply don't care enough about you because you don't fit into their pattern.

This is something I experienced at a very young age after the disease started. I never fit into any pattern that young boys found attractive. That could have also been linked to my personality, of course, but my size definitely had an impact on their decision not to date me or choose me and to go for the girls with the normal legs who fit into their pattern of how girls should be.

When you are young, you do not understand the ways teenage boys behave, and you simply feel like an alien who does not belong in any box. In fact, lipedema got me my own box that is way better than any overcrowded box. Looking back, it saved me from a few unhealthy relationships, and I might not have developed the way I did if I had fit into that pattern back then.

There are many ways that society discriminates against women with lipedema. Lipedema has an impact on our careers. As the British poll (2014) showed, 51 percent of lipedema patients reported that the disease had an impact on their ability to carry out their chosen careers, commonly citing a lack of mobility, discomfort, and inability to stand. Thirty-nine percent of lipedema patients stated that they felt restricted in their choice of careers due to the disease.

One of the biggest problems in dealing with the disease in my opinion is that once you get diagnosed and live with the certainty that you are not just too lazy and lack discipline, you have to come to terms with the word "disease."

Let me give you an example. How do you tell a person she or he is sick? It is not her fault her legs and arms look oversize in relation to the rest of her body. How do you approach someone with that knowledge without offending her and, in the same moment, try to support her? As doctors, we do it every day. We have to be committed to our patients and find the right words to tell them bad news, but in the same sentence, we have to encourage them not to give up and assure them we will help them the best we can.

As a doctor and patient, I am aiming to help people by sharing the knowledge I have gained over the last few years and offering my emotional support because I know how it feels to be in their place. In a way, this book is my attempt to be an emotional support for those who have already been diagnosed, and it is a guidebook for those who have been suspicious that something is wrong but are not aware of the real problem yet.

I see a lot of people on the streets about whom I think, *Hey, I think she has lipedema*, and I wonder whether she already knows or not. Secondly, I wonder if I should approach her and tell her. Since I cannot approach everyone, this book is my way of offering advice.

Regarding exercise, I recommend keeping yourself stretched and active as much as possible. Running a marathon won't stop your calves and ankles from being "cankles," and be careful about cardio workouts. A lot of lipedema patients complain about pain during high-intensity exercising and swelling of the legs when exercising without wearing compression garments. So please try to eat healthily and work out as much as you feel is possible for you.

I was in very good shape in my younger years until my twenties, when I stopped working out on a regular basis mostly because I got so depressed and ashamed of hitting the gym because of my lipedema legs. When I started another attempt in my late twenties, I hired a personal trainer. There was no effect, despite my working out on a regular basis and spending a lot of money on a personal trainer. That was when I decided on surgery, lying on the floor of the gym, exhausted to the limit and unable to bear the sight of my bruised and heavy limbs in the mirror any longer.

Chapter 6
How to Treat It

A little science estranges man from God, but much science leads them back to Him.

- Louis Pasteur

I really love my job, and I am used to working long hours and putting a lot of effort into it. That was not what felt wrong. In a way, my job was the only thing that felt normal to me. That saved me. I felt that there was something else I had to change. But nothing ever really changed. Then one day, I read a quote from Mahatma Gandhi that made me stumble and think: "Be the change that you wish to see in the world." Suddenly I knew that if I were not going to get up and try to change something and find a solution for my problem, life would never change the way I always wished for it to.

I dare to compare lipedema to have a benign tumor-like behavior. Both are growing without a stop. Both cannot be stopped by any other than intervention. Both love sugar. Starving the cells while getting into ketosis and sugar restriction might help. Both have to be removed surgically, and once this is done, both are gone. Lipedema is like a benign tumor.

One of the most important things I want to state here is that the sooner you undergo liposuction and a complete removal of the diseased fat tissue, the better. Some lipedema specialists recommend their patients to try conservative therapy first. Therefore wearing compression garment (class II-III) and manual lymphatic drainage is recommended.

I learned about several cases of lipedema patients in which compression of the legs and the swollen tissue did not provide comfort. They did not benefit from compression and could not even wear the garments for a single hour because of the increased pressure and pain. In my case, compression was crucial in summer and when standing for long hours. There is a special compression garment for lipedema and lymphedema called a flat-knit compression garment. It tends to be more supportive for lymphatic vessels compared to others, but it is not necessary and mandatory for every lipedema patient.

All I ever longed for was to be healthy and lead a normal life, seeing summer as just another season and not as an inevitable threat that eventually approached each year. I wanted to wear skirts and boots. My calves were so big in diameter (forty-three centimeters each) that I did not fit into any boots.

One of the first things I did after my first surgery was try on the boots I had purchased over a year before as a motivation to lose weight (how silly, I know) and that I had never fit in. They were too big. My calves' diameters were now thirty-two centimeters at the biggest point. I gave the boots to a friend of mine who had normal calves and fit in perfectly. So that was one of the moments after surgery I will never forget. I was crawling out of bed, hardly able to move and only wearing my postoperative compression garment, rummaging around my wardrobe, looking for these boots. When I tried them on, the feeling was so overwhelming that I started crying. I was so happy. It was like I had found my real calves again. I never could have imagined the liberation deriving from such a liposuction. That very moment I realized it would be worth going through three of these surgeries. I felt I could do this. And even if I could not I had to.

After my second surgery my thigh circumference had reduced ten centimeters (4 inches) on each side at the widest circumference. I fit perfectly into a size 4-6 (US) again. My intention was to change. Nobody can imagine how painful lipedema feels. You have to fight every day and you cannot give in. You always have to remember that it is a disease and not who you really are. It is so exhausting to fight it, but it is even more exhausting to live a life with lipedema. And I knew that this transition was not about becoming someone better, but about finally allowing myself to become who I had always truly meant to be.

I have seen many lipedema patients coming to our clinic at a very late stage. The only conservative treatments they had received were compression garments and many sessions of lymphatic drainages. They had already developed lip-lymphedema and lip sclerosis, which normally develops after one or two decades of suffering from lipedema. That is why I strongly recommend treating lipedema surgically at an early stage.

In our recent survey in 2017, we asked over two hundred lipedema patients who had already been operated on how painful their legs had been before liposuction (on a scale from one to ten with ten being the worst) and how much pain they sensed after the liposuction. The study showed a significant result: the mean pain was rated seventy-five on a scale of one hundred before surgery and ten out of one hundred after surgery. So my personal experience is not just a single case but also the average outcome after lipedema treatment via liposuction.[18]

Again, it is quite comparable to removing a growing benign tumor surgically. Once it is gone, it won't come back to a very high percentage and your symptoms will be gone.[6]

A lot of discussion has been going on for years, especially when it comes to insurance companies and their reluctance to cover the costs for lipedema liposuction. To sum it up, there is still a whole lot of people doubting liposuction is the best treatment to cure lipedema. To date in Germany, there are several lipedema patients suing their insurance companies, as liposuctions are expensive and can cost up to ten thousand dollars each surgery.

I was lucky enough to have parents who lent me the money. I don't want to elaborate on the German health-care and insurance systems, but I really hope that someday we will make insurance companies finally respect lipedema women and pay for their treatment. This is something I will definitely fight for, so younger generations of lipedema patients won't have to worry about how they are going to pay for their treatment.

Having undergone three maximum liposuctions in twelve months, I advise you to find a lipedema specialist. I underwent a minor liposuction of the lateral thigh regions in 2011 under local anesthesia, and I had zero benefit from it. The doctor removed less than one liter of fat from my thighs, and I had the feeling it had come back. So the crucial thing about lipedema liposuction is that the surgeon uses a very fine and blunt cannula (about three to five millimeters) when performing tumescent liposuction in the affected areas and removes every inch of diseased lipedema fat meticulously.

Once I read about a doctor who stated he did not favor liposuction for lipedema patients, as there is a high risk of postoperative lymphedema. Well, there might be a small chance or risk of injuring lymphatic vessels during the procedure, but in the overwhelming majority, it is a very unlikely event. The best thing you can do to prevent it is to find a lipedema specialist who is experienced with lipedema liposuction.

Speaking from the perspective of a doctor, I'd say it is important to be careful about the tender lymphatic vessels, and therefore, liposuction techniques for lipedema should follow longitudinal movements parallel to vessels and the lymphatic system in order to spare them. Another difference between lipedema liposuction and normal liposuction is that the former is performed around the whole circumference of the legs to remove all of the diseased fat.

I have met several fellow lipedema patients who had "normal" liposuctions done, just like me before, without any impact. That's why I emphasize that finding the right doctor and a real lipedema surgery expert is so crucial for the outcome. Secondly, I want you to know that these liposuctions are not comparable to cosmetic liposuctions. Most people do not understand that these surgeries are performed under general anesthesia and take several hours.

I have seen a lot of patients who jump out of bed two hours after rhinoplasty (nose job) or facelift patients who get on a plane to fly back home the next day after surgery. Being a plastic and aesthetic surgeon, I have performed several liposuctions myself, and I thought I knew what was coming for me. But, ladies, I was so wrong. I never could have imagined the maximum impact these lipedema liposuctions would have on my body. First of all, the doctor removed more fat than in normal patients who aim to get a little bit of thigh fat removed with liposuction. The amount of fat that gets removed in one session varies from four liters up to ten. These are maximum liposuctions, and every patient is different. A doctor has to decide individually with every patient how much sick fat can be removed in each session.

As for the postoperative phase, it is important to mention that your circulatory system will be bothered for at least two to ten days. I suffered from severe hypotonia (low blood pressure); I fainted or felt dizzy when I got up in the first two weeks. I had lost a considerable amount of blood, too, so my iron levels and hemoglobin levels were really low. Imagine: my lower body had lost 7.5 liters of fat in one session and ten liters in the second. My arms lost over four liters of pure sick lipedema fat. But these are just numbers. Keep in mind that I am a big woman (I am almost five-foot-nine), and there was a lot of diseased fat covering my legs. I had typical "cankles," and each of my lower legs had 2.5 liters of pure sick fat in it.

When my surgeon told me after the surgery, I did not believe him at first. I saw the small lower legs, and my brain was confused. It took me several days to adjust to the picture I saw when looking down. My body image had changed completely over the years. What I saw now was hardly the body I was used to, but it seemed more like the body that had been uncovered.

After tumescent liposuction it is normal that your body leaks the remaining tumescent fluid and wound fluid from the incision wholes in the skin. So the first three days I had to sleep with double sheet blankets and I can tell you it was not so much fun. You are not allowed to remove the postoperative compression garments for 6 weeks and you have to wear it days and nights. The first shower was not so easy to handle because of the dried wound fluid and the overall postoperative tissue swelling. That's why lymphatic drainage is crucial when it comes to lymphatic diseases and it is wonderful for postoperative lipedema liposuction patients.

We really do benefit from the drainage effect as conservative therapy in my opinion, but its benefits are mostly limited to a time of around twenty-four hours. Don't be surprised if you don't experience long-lasting results. Many lipedema patients have lymphatic drainage up to three times per week. I'm just emphasizing this, as general practitioners and health-care insurers often prescribe and recommend it. In my case, I kind of liked the relief it gave me after my liposuctions.

Another recommendation I can give is that swimming has almost the same beneficial effect on the lipedema swelling as lymphatic drainage. But as I said before liposuctions I could not bear the public swimming pools and felt often too ashamed to go swimming.

As I mentioned before, choose the right doctor, and he or she will choose the right treatment for you. Every lipedema patient I met was different from the others. Some needed only one or two sessions of liposuctions, others up to seven surgeries. It depends not only on your age and health status but also on the stage and grade of the disease.

Please stop listening to people who say it is not curable because there are long-term studies and clinical trials as I mentioned some of them above[18] that have examined long-term follow-up patients without recurrence of lipedema.

One of our ongoing studies examines hormone levels of fifty lipedema patients before surgery compared to three months after their last lipedema surgery. Our aim is to evaluate whether the hormone levels are changing after removal of the sick fat. My hypothesis is that the sick fat cells produce the wrong concentration of hormones, as fat tissue acts as an endocrine organ itself. It thus could have dramatic effects on the central hormone system and consequently on fertility.

Of course, a genetic disposition will always remain, and everybody is an individual human being, so there might be exceptions. But to a very high percentage, the lipedema fat does not return to the places where it has been removed via liposuction. In my case I was so worried about the disease coming back that after I had fully healed I started measuring my calves and thighs every week and to keep record. But thank god it had stayed the same size since then. I cannot emphasize enough how important it is to find a lipedema liposuction specialist to get the job done.

Eight to ten weeks after surgery, you will recognize that there is still swelling and numbness in your legs, but there will be a relief from pain and pressure pain. Moreover, you will realize—depending on the stage of lipedema you have suffered from—that your clothes will be too big. In my case, I have dropped at least three sizes. I went from a size 12 (US) back to a size 4-6 (US).

So it is a major change for the brain to adjust, as you will see. The brain has to adjust to your new body image when you look in the mirror and to the fact that there is no more neuronal sensation of pain coming from your legs. Here is my tip for you to better adjust and find yourself during this healing and regeneration phase: take pictures of your body every weekend and look at them every now and then. It helps you enormously to come to terms with your new body image.

Another advice: Don't weigh yourself immediately after surgery. There will be a lot of fluid in the wound site between the subcutaneous skin and the muscles. Weight will be of secondary importance, trust me.

Lipedema surgery is not primarily a weight-loss or aesthetic surgery. The merits are, first of all, that you won't feel pain anymore and that you will feel eager to start running again like a little child. Second, I consider it a body shaping surgery. It simply reshapes your whole appearance and you will look healthier again. I did not undergo surgery because I was keen on winning a first prize at a beauty pageant, nor did I have any aspirations for seeking love from a man I could not have had before. The reason I wanted to jump onto the operating table was that I just wanted that sick fat to be removed from my body. I wanted to get the fat suit finally unzipped. It is very hard to describe what pressure you feel that you are accepting all risks and possible adverse side effects of these surgeries.

Chapter 7

How to Heal Yourself

Natural forces within us are the true healers of disease.

- Hippocrates

Do not believe people who tell you to accept the way you look because your mother or sister or grandmother looked the same as you do. Their tree trunk legs must not be your legs any longer. It is because they might be sick, too, and they did not have the possibility of receiving a proper diagnostic process and treatment procedure. You are unique, and you have to learn to trust yourself more than everybody else.

Another very important lesson I had to learn is that you need to become your best friend. A problem that roots deep within us is that we kind of detest our bodies so much on a subconscious level. It is hard for us to even accept ourselves and, moreover, to love ourselves. Some might avoid every mirror they pass because they cannot bear their appearances. In the British poll, 86 percent of women reported low self-esteem. I always had kind of a horror moment when somebody wanted to take a picture, so I instantly offered to take the picture; that's why there are not so many existing pictures of my teenage years and adolescence. In a way, my brain started neglecting the whole lipedema fat situation. It was after my first liposuction that I started reconnecting with my body again.

As you have experienced so much despair and self-doubt/self-hatred, you will start to appreciate and love yourself again. As a woman with lipedema, you have probably completely forgotten how to love yourself, as there is a kind of invisible rupture in your mind. You somehow bisected your personality into one part ego and one part body. This body does not really belong to you, but society tells you that it is your responsibility to take care of yourself and this body.

What society does not know is that you lost your identification with this body long ago, as you lost control over your fat cells long ago. They don't belong to you in a way. No matter how much you starve yourself, they are still sitting there, laughing about you. No matter how much exercise you do, how much effort you put into yourself to make it work, you will fail. And these failures over and over again damage your self-esteem, self-worth, and confidence. In a way, it is a form of self-destruction at its most sublime level.

As soon as you accept that these past failed attempts are not your fault, you will be able to heal. If you already had surgery, your scars will heal, and so will your inner self. It takes a lot of time. Do not expect it to happen overnight, please. It is not possible to overcome all these complex traumas in one night. Give yourself a break. Breathe and be happy. You made it. You were chosen by destiny to struggle with this disease, and you managed to dismantle yourself from loads of fat that does not belong to you and never did.

Be appreciative of that. You will recognize that the real healing process starts after the wounds have closed and the scars become almost invisible. The biggest wounds are within you.

Let me give you a comparison: Let's say you had an accident with your bike, and your leg got injured, and your back was scratched up. You put a plaster on the back and focus on the leg because you see it and everybody does and because it is the obvious wound. After your leg has fully healed and you can walk again, one day you remember that there is still a Band-Aid on your back. You turn toward a mirror and rip the Band-Aid off. What you discover is a much bigger wound, and you can hardly breathe because it is so big in size that it takes your breath away. You ask yourself how you could have missed such a prominent wound, and you know that this will take some time, tender loving care, and wound dressings to completely heal.

I think you know what I want to tell you with this allegory: The leg is the body, the obvious sick fat tissue that causes trouble and can easily be removed with liposuction. The back is the soul. We know it is there, and it might have gotten injured as well, but we don't pay attention to it because we can't see it without a mirror.

This book is your mirror. Please notice that there is a wound on the back, too: your injured soul. Self-esteem must be rebuilt, and a transformation in a double sense is needed to fully heal lipedema. The transformation from a size 10 to a size 4 is one thing. People will look at you, and men will compliment you on your great looks. But the real transformation takes place inside you, my dear, from self-hatred to self-love. We are all looking for self-love because this is the only form of unconditional love we can control. Moreover, we do not even need to control it; as soon as it has developed, it will be always there. You won't need people around you who tell you every day how beautiful you look. It is nice for your ego, but that's not the reward for defeating lipedema. The true and highest reward is unconditional self-love and humbleness.

An interesting effect I came to know after I started to speak about my disease and my battle I fought was that my male friends suddenly became aware of the fact that other girls actually can have large and disproportioned legs due to lipedema, too.

They told me weeks or months later that something had changed in their perception because of my story. I felt honored and proud because I had given the guys more appreciation for women with lipedema and I had uplifted lipedema girls silently. When the guys walked through the streets or looked through photographs of girls now they had a different perspective on their bodies and did not see them as "fat" anymore, but more like "oh she probably has lipedema". When I first heard about that from a friend of mine I was so moved and I knew that I was doing something right by stepping out telling my story.

It takes a village to change society's prejudices but it takes only one girl to contribute to each other's understanding and comfort. To speak and think more gently about each other and to reduce judgmental opinions has become a wonderful mission to me.

Chapter 8
Reconciliation

Reconciliation always brings a springtime to the soul.

\- Frère Roger

After suffering from lipedema why would you need reconciliation and with whom? What is reconciliation anyway? Regarding my own experiences with lipedema it is an extremely overwhelming feeling to be freed from this diseased fat that made your life so hard and dark sometimes. Looking back you might find years of despair, self-hatred and also feelings of anger against other people who failed you. They mistook your lipedema legs for your character and you were hurt a thousands times by their comments. These negative emotions in a way poisoned your mind.

And it is time to let go of them. Let go of the resistance and vengeance you might have for them inside. If you are directing your thoughts towards powerlessness you are seeking vengeance by holding on to your feeling of powerlessness. The truth is that you have been adapted so long to this emotional state of powerlessness that you have made this feeling a splendid companion of yours. Once your "problem" is solved you are still in company of this feeling, although it is not needed anymore. So I found it very helpful to acknowledge that this strong emotion was there and I was grateful for it. You never know how things might have turned out if it was not for this hopelessness I had to overcome during my time with lipedema.

On a more abstract level you may find it interesting that you got to suffer from lipedema in the first place. It is like I described a heavy suit of fat. Fat tissue is basically one of the most important tissues in our bodies. It keeps us warm, protects us and restores a lot of energy. So why do we store massive amounts of fat cells that we cannot get rid of in any normal sense? Maybe we want to protect ourselves from the outer world unconsciously because we are very sensitive people or because we have experienced trauma. As I am not a psychiatrist and neither a spiritual healer in any sense, I just like to illuminate this disease from every possible angle.

After lipedema surgeries there will be a wide range of positive feelings popping up such as joy, happiness, relief and freedom. I experienced all these very positive feelings and I felt so blessed everyday I put on my new trousers, my new boots or any other kind of clothing that I had not been able to wear for so many years. I had an immediate relief of pain in my legs and arms and I gained incredible strength after surgeries, although they exhausted me in the beginning very much. And still I felt that there was a kind of insecurity and fear within me.

My worries included fears like: Will the fat come back? What if this is only borrowed heaven? Maybe I will suffer from lipedema in the future after hormonal changes again? What should I do to prevent it from coming back? All these nagging thoughts were still with me because I had not given up to the feeling of powerlessness yet. I was still in a state of resistance. I could not trust the cease-fire yet. I could not believe that the fight was over and that I had won the battle.

From now on I could do the same equation with weight gain and weight loss like everybody else did, but I could not trust myself. I had been living with distrust all these years and as I described prior it had begun to be part of my emotional companions everyday. Insecurity and self-distrust come with a lack of self-confidence and bring up self-worth issues. So instead of letting distrust and insecurity go, I just put them onto another topic. Now I was not worried about losing weight or how to get rid of the disease, now I was worried constantly about what if it came back one day?

It took me several months after my last surgery when I realized that my lipedema fat had not come back in the course of one and a half years and that my measurements were still the same except for my breasts, they had increased in volume. I came to the conclusion that fear had been my companion for long enough time and I was ready to let it go. I felt like I was too young to worry all my life about lipedema. Instead, I could focus on so many positive things and that it was time for an emotional detox.

By building a deeper connection to yourself you realize that the power you hold within yourself and faith in yourself is far bigger than any powerlessness or self-distrust. As I am a medical doctor and scientist I always try to think in an analytic way and to find reasonable questions and explanations.

The theory of reconciliation and healing your emotional wounds is nothing that interferes with my lifelong scientific approach. In contrary, exploring my feelings and working with them for the first time gave me more sense and peace than I had ever experienced before. If you are in the same situation as me and are affected by lipedema from young adolescence on, you might have been – just as me- unable to build up a safe emotional connection to yourself and your body.

As in my case the start of lipedema followed shortly after puberty I did not understand that it was two different things that happened in a short period of time. A lack of self-confidence due to body issues is interfering with the adolescent age of discovering and creating identity. This was a lesson I had to understand before I could move on. I had to forgive myself. For not trusting myself, for shaming myself and blaming me for a lack of self-discipline everyone else seemed to have except for me. I had to forgive others who blamed me without better knowing lipedema and I had to let go of the permanent fear lipedema would come back one day.

As fear is described as the opposite emotion of love, some of you might just state – let's love yourself and fear will vanish. But how do you learn to love yourself after years of negative body imaging and self-hatred? How can you escape the vicious circle? It starts with forgiveness. Reconciliation. When you start to let go of shaming and accept that it is not your fault and never was, you will feel a sudden relief of pain. This can take a long time and is not easy to accomplish. You might not be able to relate to that before you had your surgeries done. But it is something very rewarding you should try. The real work is waiting for you on the inside.

Chapter 9
My Lipedema Diet

Your body is your temple.
Keep it pure and clean for the soul to reside in.

\- B.K.S. Iyengar

Having undergone a total of three maximum lipedema liposuctions, I experienced relief from pressure pain; swelling and it gave me a new body image. In a way, it was a revelation. I felt a thousand times more self-confident, and shopping for clothes did not give me rashes anymore. Finally I was able to start exercising again, due to my increased mobility and I could stand in surgery for many hours without feeling lipedema pain. But after the scars had healed and the postoperative swelling was gone and I got back to my normal, everyday life I still had one problem to solve: What should I eat? Should I go on a special diet? What if it all came back?

One of my biggest problems I faced after my third lipedema surgery was that my overall swelling had not reduced to the extent I had wished upon. So what I mean was that my cheeks were still "swollen" and so were my belly and hands. I had lost almost 20 lbs initially after the final surgery but gained back 9 lbs somehow afterwards when I indulged on sweets, carbohydrates and did not exercise regularly due to long working hours.

For a long time I had thought that after the last lipedema surgery my body would completely go back to normal, but I learned that there was still one problem left. The diseased fat had been removed and did not come back in the areas that had been surgically treated. It gave me incredible mobility and pain had simply vanished. But the puffy swelling and the weight gain in other areas of my body did not contribute to my happiness. As I mentioned before I became a board certified doctor of the German society for nutrition. I tried to figure out what made me swell and if there was a kind of nutrition I could adapt in order to reduce swelling and weight gain in lipedema.

I learned that a lot of products aggravate swelling and in fact the list of what will make you not feel good is very long. An important thing to know about foods that can cause swelling and enhance edema in general is high sodium consumption. Sodium intake should be limited to 2,300 mg per day according to Mayo Clinic references. Moreover the influence of sodium and potassium intake and insulin resistance on blood pressure in healthy normotensive individuals is more evident in women than men.[20]

Another scientist recently published a paper where they could show that tissue sodium content is elevated in the skin and subcutaneous adipose tissue in women with lipedema.[21]

So by the law of osmosis water follows sodium into the tissue and therefore we need to reduce sodium intake in our nutrition to reduce water leaking trough the vessels and therefore reduce the painful swelling.

What makes you swell and bloat may vary individually, but I realized that processed grains such as commercial pancakes, waffles, salty snack crackers and any sort of ready-to-eat-food worsened swelling. Either I am gluten-sensitive additionally to lipedema or it is a coincidence yet to be further investigated. The real celiac disease usually occurs in children at a very young age presenting with flatulence, nausea, stomach pains, and lack of appetite, chronic diarrhea resulting in growth impairment.[22]

So I started to learn more about our lymphatic gut system and how the uptake of different kinds of oil can have an impact on the amount of produced lymph fluid. Did you know the gut plays a huge part in the lymphatic system? For example leaky lymphatics can be influenced by food intake that act anti-inflammatory.

L-Arginine is a semi-essential amino acid that contributes to healthy vessels and is reduced in inflammatory diseases.[23] For example sources of L-arginine are eggs, lentils, nuts and food rich in nitrate/nitrite are leafy greens.

What is an anti-inflammatory nutrition anyway? We all know inflammation on the surface of the skin is characterized by local redness, heat, swelling and pain. Inflammation is not basically a bad thing. In contrary - it is the cornerstone of the body's healing response. Wound healing would be impossible without an inflammatory response of the body. So to say, inflammation is action.

Our immune system initializes a very old orchestration of factors that can change something in your body. But when inflammation persists or serves no purpose, it damages the body and causes illness. Therefore it is well known that stress, lack of exercise, genetic predisposition, and exposure to toxins can all contribute to such chronic inflammation, but dietary choices play a big role as well. There have been several attempts by nutritionists to define a distinctive "anti-inflammatory diet" which is simply put a very clean and healthy way of eating. Still you will find that there are grains and many carbs in the recommendations that I simply cannot worship for my lipedema diet.

Repair and renovation work is required in every cell at all times. The old cells die off and are replaced by new ones. This is the basis for maintaining the structure and function of the entire body. And for this repair work, building materials are needed, similar to building houses. Most of the building materials can be made by the body itself, but not by so-called essential nutrients, e.g. essential amino acids and essential fatty acids. These must be absorbed by food.

To my disappointment I mostly found recommendations about what I should *not* eat when I was suffering from lipedema, and that was quite a list. So my intention was to find out about *what* I could eat.

My strong interest in nutrition definitely roots in my history of suffering for ten years from the disease, which let me try every fancy diet. From low fat to vegan and paleo, I tried everything. Even formula diets that made me lose ten pounds of water weight, but as soon as I started eating solid food, I gained back every lost pound. I remember a time when my meals consisted of a protein shake and a handful of almonds. Like many other lipedema patients, I starved myself. I was tired and undernourished but still "fat." This was one of the most ridiculous things I could imagine. But when I compared my experiences to other lipedema patients, they told me they had experienced the same thing. As lipedema patients, we are often perceived by society as lazy and lacking in discipline. I think the truth is that most lipedema patients are extremely disciplined and are falsely accused of the opposite.

After my last surgery I started a lipedema nutrition diary. I called it "mylipedemadiet". What I found super annoying with all the other pre-existing diet plans was that they provided a fixed meal plan where you had to rigorously stick to and if you did one thing differently and it did not have the successful outcome – you failed. Again. And it was not the diet but your fault again, because you did not have the discipline to follow through. Others merely provided long lists of food – part of those I had never heard of before and my brain simply faced too many choices. When you have lipedema or after lipedema surgeries you can get frustrated from time to time because you are facing weight gain and want to put a bar in front of it.

With the help of understanding the basic form of what to eat, you will be positively energized and easily follow your instinct. I truly believe in thinking positive. Thinking about all the things you are not allowed to eat and you have to avoid can be so exhausting and emotionally depressing. So we will focus on what to eat. Negative imperatives have probably tortured our subconscious for many years. You should avoid eating carbs. You should not eat sweets. You should stay away from coffee and tea. I could go on for pages and pages, and I won't do the same. Instead you could make a list of things you *should* eat, and the next time you are wandering through a supermarket, you will notice that you might have some appetite for broccoli and feta cheese and pineapples for dinner because your brain has connected the positive dots between—this is good for my body, and this is what I want to eat. It is so much harder for your brain to remember what is on the list that you cannot eat, compared to when you have a list of what you should eat. We have to focus on the positive aspects in life and also in our nutrition.

According to many lipedema women sharing their stories on Facebook[TM], the way of a ketogenic diet provides relief of pain, reduces swelling, and helps to lose weight overall. A ketogenic diet is based on a very low-carb and high-fat diet. They receive 60 to 75 percent of their calories from fat, 15 to 30 percent from protein, and the rest from carbohydrates, mostly contained in vegetables.[24]

One explanation possible, therefore, could be the absence of sugar (glucose or saccharides to be more specific) in your diet. Scientists have found out that a ketogenic diet can be anti-inflammatory and good for tumor patients to stop the tumor from growing.[25]

Once more my lipedema tumor-like theory could be backed. If you feed a tumor with sugar, it will do what it can do best—grow. The experience seems to be the same with lipedema fat tissue—it is constantly, progressively growing over the years. Once you cut the carbs, you will go into the state of ketosis and will realize a certain kind of relief.

But if it is so easy—just cut the carbs and go into ketosis (burning fat with fat, receiving energy only from ketone bodies, a substrate made from fat)—lipedema could be healed in every woman within a few weeks or months, no? Well, you already know the answer. It is not that easy. I have read many success stories on "keto blogs" from lipedema patients, and many of them really described a dramatic loss of weight and a relief in pain and swelling reduction. But it seemed from their pictures that their typical lipedema shape of calves and thighs had not changed.

In my opinion, the diet is quite controversial and you have to start over all again once you get off track and indulge in a bagel. In my opinion, this is not a desirable plan to stick to for the rest of my life. But I got further interested in the topic and it lead me to pursue my quest in finding my ideal lipedema diet. I was looking for a plan that I could lose 20 lbs of weight and stay slim despite leading a busy and productive life as a plastic surgeon.

German guidelines for nutrition still recommend a total energy intake to be deriving 60% of carbohydrates, which is way too high for lipedema patients in my opinion. At that point, I have to say I believe that a ketogenic diet can be helpful for lipedema patients if they like eating high-fat foods and can live with the downsides of this diet (e.g., halitosis or the bad smell of the mouth due to ketone bodies like acetone).

Nevertheless high-fat diets have been shown to accelerate cognitive impairment like Alzheimer's disease in mice.[26] Although a low-calorie ketogenic diet for weight loss seems to be safe for a short term of twenty-one days, the long-term results of a life-long ketogenic diet have not been evaluated yet.[24] In my opinion, what makes the difference for lipedema is a very low proportion of carbs that has a positive impact on the lipedema disease and reduces symptoms the ketogenic way of eating does.

I believe the tricky thing about finding the right nutrition and diet for lipedema patients is that our metabolism acts completely different from the average person. One of the fundamental research questions is whether the diseased fat pads have direct influence and consequences for our metabolism or not. So maybe our genetic background stays the same even after having undergone lipedema liposuction and we still have to face different metabolic challenges compared to other women? One major problem is the fact that we might be more prone to have experienced eating disorders in the past.

In the British survey, 45 percent of lipedema patients reported that they were suffering from an eating disorder, and I had times when I simply did not care about what I ate because I was so desperate. I believe as a lipedema patient, it is easy to be well educated about food and still lose any relation to it, as you cannot experience the same laws of physics and energy that seem to work with every other human being around you. Even if you lose overall weight, you never lose it at the lipedema zones.

In my opinion every meal of a successful long lasting diet contains fibers, greens, fat and protein. I aimed to go for a high-protein, low-carb, and medium fat diet, stating that this has a better chance of providing a feasible, life-long form of nutrition. I prefer nutrition high in protein (60-70%), moderate in fat (20-30%

best: polyunsaturated fatty acids, PUFA), and low carbohydrates (10%). The main reason for this is that the body must burn energy solely for utilization of proteins. Moreover, there is no muscle-wasting as long as you provide your body with high-protein nutrition, and satiety settles in sooner.

Studies have shown that dietary carbohydrate restriction improves insulin sensitivity, high blood pressure, microvascular function and cellular adhesion markers in individuals suffering from metabolic disorders.[27]

Fat is not something to avoid. Fat is essential for normal growth and development and also provides energy, protects our organs, maintains cell membranes, and helps the body absorb and process nutrients. Even better, it helps the body to burn restored fat.

50 years ago scientists found that saturated fatty acids, raised LDL (low density lipoprotein) cholesterol levels. So-called "low fat" diets were favored.

A few "low fat" decades later we face a growing problem with obesity in Western countries and opinions have changed as research has once more investigated the up and down sides of fat. Many nutrients including vitamins A, D, E, and K are fat-soluble, meaning that the body can't absorb them without fat. If your body isn't absorbing nutrients properly, that can lead to vitamin deficiencies and bring on dry skin, blindness, brittle bones, muscle pains, and abnormal blood clotting.[28]

Preferable foods (like fish, seeds, nuts, leafy vegetables, olive oil, and of course, avocados) pack tons of vitamins and nutrients. This is one of my fundamental beliefs from what I have experienced during my search for my perfect satisfying long lasting lipedema diet.

From my experience of the main reasons for weight loss in lipedema diet is that you work with anti-inflammatory and anti swelling foods. The reason why anti-inflammatory foods are favorable might be because the sick fat cells are surrounded by inflammatory cells which cause secondary fibrosis in the fat tissue.[15] In higher stages of lipedema you see a typical fibrosclerosis within the fat tissue, that's when fat cells have been surrounded by inflammatory cells like walls of brick.

There are several foods that can reduce inflammation and help you dissolve the walls of bricks around your fat cells. Nutrition rich in polyphenols can reduce the formation of free radicals in the body, protecting cells and molecules from damage.[29] These free radicals are known to play a role in aging and all sorts of diseases. For example EGCG (Epigallocatechin Gallate) is one of the most powerful compounds in green tea. It has been studied to treat various diseases and may be one of the main reasons green tea has such powerful medicinal effects.[29]

A lot of people ask me about the benefits of intermittent fasting. How does losing weight with interval fasting work? The principle is very simple: in the 16 hours when you are not eating any food your insulin levels will drop. In this insulin break, your body can go to the fat stores and release the energy stored there to use them. Study participants even report improved sleeping patterns and more ability to concentrate throughout the day because they adjusted their eating habits to the rhythm of the 08/16.[30]

It means that you are allowed to eat for 8 hours a day and can eat two or three meals a day. The remaining 16 hours you fast and consume only calorie-free drinks. I am trying to stick to 08/16 and intermittent fasting and I sleep better since that.

I start my day with a cup of green tea and eat as much protein as possible—for example, yogurt, eggs, salmon or nuts. I try to eat fish (rich in omega-3 fatty acids) at least twice a week and avoid highly processed, overly greasy, and super sweet foods.

As hard as it is but I avoid pastries by all means, as they contain a lot of trans fatty acids, and a lot of lipedema friends also find that they get heavily bloated when eating cake and bread. Chose whole grains if you cannot live without bread but try to substitute your breakfast toast with a bowl of yogurt with a handful of blueberries, for example. I could notice the difference immediately after a few days.

It is not about interdictions. Nobody can live forever without ever eating a piece of cake, chocolate, or bread from time to time. We are human. But the more often you choose correctly for your body, the better it is for you. Every time you pass by a bakery, you can choose. Think about it. Life is mostly about choices. Start making the right ones more often than the wrongs; then nothing is forever prohibited. In a world full of choices it is even harder to choose wisely all the time.

Many foods have been integrated in our lives from an early age on without ever giving a thought whether they are good for us or not. We are being confused by marketing strategies and thousands of professional advertisers and so called experts who claim to know what is best for us. Healthy foods have been defined by being labeled as such. Being overwhelmed by the abundance of "healthy food" you can get lost in making the right choices.

Regarding supplements, I am taking minimum 5.6 IE of vitamin D orally per week in order to ensure a normal level. In my opinion, additional substitutions of specific vitamins in healthy lipedema patients need to be further investigated before anybody can give a concrete statement or recommendation. The overall supply of vitamins and trace elements must be ensured via a healthy diet and not over pills, unless there is a specific demand for it.

From my personal experience, I believe that it is best for women with lipedema to follow an anti-inflammatory, low-carb diet. Simply put, you should focus on lean protein, leafy greens, and vegetables such as spinach, kale, broccoli, and green salad. Be careful when it comes to fruit. They contain a lot of sugar; melons, for instance, have a lot of water but also a lot of sugar. So do grapes. They taste delicious and contain resveratrol, a substance that is also found to be cardio protective and an antioxidant.[31]

But be aware that because of the amount of saccharides in grapes, you can eat the equivalent of sweet jellybeans instead. You could instead go for all types of berries: strawberries, blueberries, and gooseberries. They are rich in antioxidants and high in fiber.

Dairy should be left out in the beginning and during weight loss phases as they contain lactose, a form of sugar and for many of us it is not tolerable especially when an irritable bowel disease is co-existent.

Researchers conducted a 2010 clinical trial of irritable bowel disease (IBD) patients and found that maintaining a low-FODMAP diet reduced their symptoms. The FODMAP concept is based on the assumption that functional gastrointestinal complaints in IBD are due, among other things, to flatulence in the intestine.[32]

FODMAPs are widespread in the western diet and comprise monosaccharides (fructose), disaccharides (lactose), oligosaccharides (fructans and galactans), and polyols (alcohol) and are poorly absorbed in the small intestine. Their ingestion increases delivery of readily fermentable substrates and water to the gut, which is likely to induce luminal distension and induction of functional gut symptoms. The restriction of their intake has been shown to reduce functional gut symptoms. They thus migrate quickly into the large intestine, where bacteria ferment them. As a by-product of the fermentation process, gases, e.g. as hydrogen, are released and lead to the aforementioned complaints.[32]

My disease had led me to become a German board certified doctor for nutrition and I am currently investigating several natural substances that seem to have impact on lipid metabolism in lipedema cells. It might not be a cure comparable to radical liposuction but my goal is to understand the complex metabolism of these lipedema fat cells and to develop a supportive nutrition that enhances fat burning of lipedema cells and leads to a reduction of swelling and pain. Years of basic science will not be enough to fully understand the complexity of this disease but we can try to improve our lives in the meanwhile, right? This is my passion and why I work to reach this personal goal, not only for me but also for all who suffer from lipedema like I did.

Chapter 10

Embracing it all

My past has not defined me, destroyed me, deterred me, or defeated me; it has only strengthened me.

- Dr. Steve Maraboli

The story of lipedema seems to be a story of darkness. There is a saying that only the ones who have experienced darkness can appreciate light. I believe that is true.

As I mentioned before, you will not be the same person after your surgeries and your struggle with fighting lipedema. I was so absorbed by my disease throughout all these years, trying to survive summer by summer and trying to find happiness in material things and my career, that I did not feel that my relationship with myself had become sicker and sicker. But it was the change I had always prayed for. I prayed to God to give me the strength to meet my destiny. You have to be very careful what you pray for. I did not really know what to expect from this prayer. But it was a prayer I said over and over again, and it came from my deepest self. So God gave me hard times to grow stronger, and he let me discover my fate. I never thought I had a real disease.

Like I said, life is about choices. I chose myself. I chose to find my true self and to live life to the fullest by fighting for the body that belonged to me. I can tell you it is hard, and you will have very dark moments of despair and doubt. But it was worth it all the way. By dissolving every old structure of who I was and breaking down my walls, my old ego was finally collapsing, and I could breathe again.

One of the first things I remember after lipedema surgery was that, to my surprise, I did not have any pain. I did not have pain from the surgery because it was so gently performed. And best of all, my constant pressure pain was simply gone. It is not a unique experience, as I listened to many other lipedema patients who reported the same thing. The surgeries were a kind of liberation. I cannot describe the moments of joy in my new every day life I experienced when I suddenly felt comfortable to wear a skirt. Long hours of standing were suddenly not painful or exhausting anymore.

This is the kind of freedom you experience after liposuction has removed all the sick fat that does not really belong to you. I suffered from postoperative swelling for quite a long time, but this was not comparable to the lipedema swelling at all. I have to say I feel sorry for all of those women who have not had the possibility to undergo liposuction yet. I pray that one day this treatment will be available for every lipedema patient and I will keep on fighting to make this disease more transparent and recognized in the medical field.

I have experienced a change in the last few months and there are more and more plastic surgeons who have become very interested and educated in the field of lipedema. Maybe we find the pathologic mechanism soon and deliver proof of a gene defect or even provide an objective a reliable blood test for lipedema, so health insurance companies will have to pay for the liposuctions. I am very thankful for the opportunities I had and for the excellent treatment I received in Germany by my marvelous surgeon and his team. After my third surgery I looked and felt like a different person. I had lost 23 liters of lipedema fat all over my body and I was able to start living a normal life again.

To me it felt like I had turned back time and finally found myself in my real skinny body. I took yoga classes again twice per week and I started running. A sport I could have never done before the surgeries due to pain and exhaustion. I once read about the so called "lipedema fatigue" meaning that lipedema patients are getting tired sooner from exercise and I suddenly felt that something was different. I think the most important step for me was to accept that the way I looked and the condition I had was not my fault.

That's why I wrote this book. I found helpful information and other lipedema friends on Facebook™ when I started looking for it but the feeling I want to share with a lot more people is to become confident again. Our mission should be to speak up for lipedema and for ourselves. We should all stand together and fight social prejudices that make us feel so weak because they merely derive from ignorance. I have started to teach medical students in my courses about lipedema emphasizing also the differences between lymphedema and lipedema and anybody can start at their neighbor's place to educate. It will take some time but I know it is worth the fight. Once you lift up your wings the freedom you experience is endless.

Chapter 11

On Becoming a Swan

*Hope is the thing with feathers, that perches in the soul
and sings the tune without words, and never stops at all.*

\- Emily Dickinson

As a plastic surgery resident, I have seen patients who are seeking perfection through cosmetic surgery. But usually they are healthy beautiful patients seeking minor corrections or improvements done by surgery or with minimal invasive approaches. With lipedema patients, it is a totally different game. When we are consulting a plastic surgeon we do not seek perfection. We cannot imagine the aesthetic outcome, and we do not know how we will look like after surgery.

I consider it somehow more of a reconstructive surgery. First of all, we have a disease of fat tissues that can be approached through a surgical procedure. Second of all, we are experiencing pain, and when the pain is gone, we are happy. It really is that simple. We are less concerned about the texture of our skin or scars. We do not care about scars. We merely seek for a surgeon who can remove as much of the diseased fat as possible. In the majority of cases more than one surgery is required. These exhausting and very expensive surgeries are not easy to handle and require a high amount of frustration tolerance, fearlessness and endurance.

There is a kind of deep satisfaction and consolation I found with my body so that I do not wish to have another body or envy other people any longer. This state of mind and satisfaction are invaluable.

Once again, this book was written for all of you who are experiencing a similar situation. Either you have doubt that something is wrong with your body and you might actually suffer from lipedema as well, or you have already been diagnosed by a doctor and feel left out and alone with moments of insecurity, despair, and doubt about yourself and what to do. Maybe you have already started the fight and have even undergone lipedema liposuction and want to compare your experiences with mine.

I am also happy if you are a relative or spouse of a lipedema patient. Your task is to support your lipedema person as much as you can. It is not really helpful if we are told, "Oh, it is not that severe, my dear," because maybe you think it is helpful if you flatter us and try to make us feel good, but it simply drives us crazy in that moment because to us it is "severe." There are many women with lipedema who do not have any support.

I was lucky enough to have one friend who supported me all the way through the darkness. Sometimes I call her a "light worker" because that is what she does. She brings light into the darkness, and you cannot compare it to anything else. Conversations with her were enlightening, and she was always encouraging me not to give up when I did not see any sense or had lost hope. She was also a big supporter of the idea of sharing my story with you and bringing my light into your world. Moreover, I am very thankful for all the people who supported me during that year while I completed those three surgeries and who took care of me after the exhausting surgeries or made my life easier.

If there were a symbol I had to choose for lipedema women, it would be a swan. In many cultures, swan symbolism has a long tradition of representing beauty, gracefulness, passion, and pure love. They are connected to the sun, and they symbolize light and all that is good. In Hinduism, swans represent the connection between the material world and the spiritual world in perfect harmony. To me, the grace of a swan is comparable to the grace of a lipedema woman. Like any other gift, the gift of grace can be yours only if you reach out and take it. Maybe being able to reach out and take it is a gift, too.

In the Celtic mind, swans were also observed in the context of movement, and they kept a promise. If a swan appeared to them, they saw the swan as a representative of the rising glory of a new day. The swan seems to be floating elegantly in the water of a lake forever. But it is not bound to that. People make the mistake of assuming they are bound to the water because that is where they see them when they first look.

But swans possess incredible abilities and strength, and they can rise to the skies and fly wherever they like. This is similar to us. People see a lipedema patient and won't give a second thought about her ability to transform. This is the real power of lipedema: the power of transformation to rise above, similar to a swan ascending from the lake to the skies from one moment to the other.

That's why I chose the title for this book. You are a swan in disguise. These layers of diseased fat cells you fought against for all these years are in fact your chance to rise. It is hard, yes. The transformation is not free, and it is not happening overnight, but once you stretch your wings and realize you were made to fly like all the other birds that you envied all the time, you will find your strength to go all the way.

There is another reason I put "swan" in the title. When I was a little girl, my mother took me to the ballet, and we watched the famous *Swan Lake*. I loved the grace and lightness the ballerinas showed onstage, and a picture of harmony and impeccable beauty emerged. But as we all know, ballet is hard work. The pain, discipline, and torment before perfect harmony can appear are well known.

In *Swan Lake*, the story is about a princess called Odette and her crowd of girls who have been jinxed into becoming swans by a sorcerer. They can only leave the lake and their swan bodies at night, and as soon as daylight touches their female bodies, they turn into swans again. Only true love can break the spell.

In the story of *Swan Lake*, a prince called Siegfried falls in love with the swan princess, Odette. But he is betrayed when the sorcerer puts a spell on his daughter so she resembles Odette, and so he swears his love to the wrong girl. Odette has to stay forever in her swan body, and her heart is broken.

The prince is devastated when he finds out he was betrayed by a sorcerer's bad trick and runs to the lake, horrified. In the end, they both drown in the lake, as they still love each other and don't see any possibility of being together in this world.

In my opinion, this story is full of analogies for the story of lipedema patients. We are sometimes mistaken and not seen because of our appearance. We might find a prince from time to time who really sees our beauty and loves us truly, but to break the spell a sorcerer has put on us, the only true love demanded is to love ourselves. We need to recognize our fate and fight it to break the curse. It might be a genetic disorder with a family history and not a sorcerer who put the spell on us. Maybe you don't have the opportunity to have all the liposuction treatments done immediately. But you can enter the transformation process as soon as you finish reading these pages. Embracing the disease is the first step, and you probably won't be able to fly immediately. The weight on your wings is too heavy, I know.

Becoming a swan requires not only faith and self-love, but also a kind of fearlessness. And I wish for you to discover your strength, your power and your fearlessness.

It took me a long way to come to write these final sentences. I have struggled for over several months to finally publish this book. As a lipedema girl I was constantly afraid to be seen in public or to speak in front of an audience, which I had to do more often than I had wished for. I did not feel comfortable and I prayed sometimes I were invisible. So nobody would stare at my legs or arms. I was afraid of myself. Fear was a constant travel companion in my life and I did not have the courage to stand up and speak up. This book is also dedicated to my fearlessness. I am not afraid anymore to be seen in public and I do not feel ashamed for my appearance or my story any more. Even if there is only one woman in this world suffering from lipedema that I will give hope with this book, all my work and courage was worth it.

Acknowledgements

I would like to thank a few people who have inspired and deeply touched me in the course of the last years while fighting lipedema.

First of all I want to thank my family who has inspired me in the first place to share my story and write this book. You helped me throughout one of the most difficult situations in my life. You picked me up from hospital after surgery, took care of me and you were the rock in my life during an important period of time.

I would like to thank my research team and collaborators for believing in our research and working long hours and inspiring me with their knowledge and experience. I am so grateful for the fighting chance the Lipedema Foundation™ gave me, not only for funding my research project and believing in a rookie but also for connecting me with the rest of the lipedema research world and its fantastic people.

Most personally I want to thank my friends who supported me during the struggle of writing and publishing. Without their helpful advice this book would have never been published.

About the Author

Anna-Theresa Bauer, MD, is a German-educated doctor specializing in plastic surgery and nutrition. Since discovering lipedema, she has become dedicated to learning more about its causes and potential treatments.

A sufferer herself, she is one of the leading scientists worldwide in the study of lipedema, finding ways to help women thrive in spite of being diagnosed with this little-known disease. Besides her experimental research investigating the pathology of lipedema she is currently creating holistic treatment options to provide patients the best medical care for lipedema available.

Reference List

[1] A.B. Halk, R.J. Damstra, First Dutch guidelines on lipedema using the international classification of functioning, disability and health, Phlebology (2016).

[2] S. Reich-Schupke, W. Schmeller, W.J. Brauer, M.E. Cornely, G. Faerber, M. Ludwig, G. Lulay, A. Miller, S. Rapprich, D.F. Richter, V. Schacht, K. Schrader, M. Stucker, C. Ure, S1 guidelines: Lipedema, Journal der Deutschen Dermatologischen Gesellschaft = Journal of the German Society of Dermatology : JDDG 15(7) (2017) 758-767.

[3] I. Forner-Cordero, G. Szolnoky, A. Forner-Cordero, L. Kemeny, Lipedema: an overview of its clinical manifestations, diagnosis and treatment of the disproportional fatty deposition syndrome - systematic review, Clin Obes 2(3-4) (2012) 86-95.

[4] E. Wenczl, J. Daroczy, [Lipedema, a barely known disease: diagnosis, associated diseases and therapy], Orv. Hetil. 149(45) (2008) 2121-7.

[5] D.W. Buck, 2nd, K.L. Herbst, Lipedema: A Relatively Common Disease with Extremely Common Misconceptions, Plastic and reconstructive surgery. Global open 4(9) (2016) e1043.

[6] A.W. Peled, S.A. Slavin, H. Brorson, Long-term Outcome After Surgical Treatment of Lipedema, Ann. Plast. Surg. 68(3) (2012) 303-7.

[7] H. Brorson, Liposuction normalizes - in contrast to other therapies - lymphedema-induced adipose tissue hypertrophy, Handchir. Mikrochir. Plast. Chir. 44(6) (2012) 348-54.

[8] A. Baumgartner, M. Hueppe, W. Schmeller, Long-term benefit of liposuction in patients with lipoedema: a follow-up study after an average of 4 and 8 years, Br. J. Dermatol. 174(5) (2016) 1061-7.

[9] W. Schmeller, M. Hueppe, I. Meier-Vollrath, Tumescent liposuction in lipoedema yields good

long-term results, Br. J. Dermatol. 166(1) (2012) 161-8.

[10] C.E. Fife, E.A. Maus, M.J. Carter, Lipedema: a frequently misdiagnosed and misunderstood fatty deposition syndrome, Advances in skin & wound care 23(2) (2010) 81-92; quiz 93-4.

[11] A.H. Child, K.D. Gordon, P. Sharpe, G. Brice, P. Ostergaard, S. Jeffery, P.S. Mortimer, Lipedema: an inherited condition, Am. J. Med. Genet. A 152a(4) (2010) 970-6.

[12] U. Langen, R. Schmitz, H. Steppuhn, [Prevalence of allergic diseases in Germany: results of the German Health Interview and Examination Survey for Adults (DEGS1)], Bundesgesundheitsblatt, Gesundheitsforschung, Gesundheitsschutz 56(5-6) (2013) 698-706.

[13] P.N. Taylor, D. Albrecht, A. Scholz, G. Gutierrez-Buey, J.H. Lazarus, C.M. Dayan, O.E. Okosieme, Global epidemiology of hyperthyroidism and hypothyroidism, Nat. Rev. Endocrinol. (2018).

[14] S. Reich-Schupke, W. Schmeller, W.J. Brauer, M.E. Cornely, G. Faerber, M. Ludwig, G. Lulay, A. Miller, S. Rapprich, D.F. Richter, V. Schacht, K. Schrader, M. Stucker, C. Ure, S1-Leitlinie Lipodem, Journal der Deutschen Dermatologischen Gesellschaft = Journal of the German Society of Dermatology : JDDG 15(7) (2017) 758-768.

[15] H. Suga, J. Araki, N. Aoi, H. Kato, T. Higashino, K. Yoshimura, Adipose tissue remodeling in lipedema: adipocyte death and concurrent regeneration, J. Cutan. Pathol. 36(12) (2009) 1293-8.

[16] G. Szolnoky, A. Nemes, H. Gavaller, T. Forster, L. Kemeny, Lipedema is associated with increased aortic stiffness, Lymphology 45(2) (2012) 71-9.

[17] S. Evans, Lipoedema: the first UK patient survey, Br. J. Community Nurs. 18(4 Suppl) (2013) S26-7.

[18] M. Dadras, P.J. Mallinger, C.C. Corterier, S. Theodosiadi, M. Ghods, Liposuction in the

Treatment of Lipedema: A Longitudinal Study, Archives of plastic surgery 44(4) (2017) 324-331.

[19] G. Szolnoky, Currently the best treatment for lipoedema, Br. J. Dermatol. 174(5) (2016) 959-60.

[20] S. Murao, Y. Takata, M. Yasuda, H. Osawa, F. Kohi, The influence of sodium and potassium intake and insulin resistance on blood pressure in normotensive individuals is more evident in women, Am. J. Hypertens. (2018).

[21] R. Crescenzi, A. Marton, P.M.C. Donahue, H.B. Mahany, S.K. Lants, P. Wang, J.A. Beckman, M.J. Donahue, J. Titze, Tissue Sodium Content is Elevated in the Skin and Subcutaneous Adipose Tissue in Women with Lipedema, Obesity (Silver Spring, Md.) 26(2) (2018) 310-317.

[22] P. Singh, A. Arora, T.A. Strand, D.A. Leffler, C. Catassi, P.H. Green, C.P. Kelly, V. Ahuja, G.K. Makharia, Global Prevalence of Celiac Disease: Systematic Review and Meta-analysis, Clin. Gastroenterol. Hepatol. (2018).

[23] D. Fukumura, F. Yuan, M. Endo, R.K. Jain, Role of nitric oxide in tumor microcirculation. Blood flow, vascular permeability, and leukocyte-endothelial interactions, Am. J. Pathol. 150(2) (1997) 713-25.

[24] C. Colica, G. Merra, A. Gasbarrini, A. De Lorenzo, G. Cioccoloni, P. Gualtieri, M.A. Perrone, S. Bernardini, V. Bernardo, L. Di Renzo, M. Marchetti, Efficacy and safety of very-low-calorie ketogenic diet: a double blind randomized crossover study, Eur. Rev. Med. Pharmacol. Sci. 21(9) (2017) 2274-2289.

[25] R.J. Klement, Beneficial effects of ketogenic diets for cancer patients: a realist review with focus on evidence and confirmation, Med. Oncol. 34(8) (2017) 132.

[26] S.K. Sah, C. Lee, J.H. Jang, G.H. Park, Effect of high-fat diet on cognitive impairment in triple-transgenic mice model of Alzheimer's disease, Biochem. Biophys. Res. Commun. (2017).

[27] K.D. Ballard, E.E. Quann, B.R. Kupchak, B.M. Volk, D.M. Kawiecki, M.L. Fernandez, R.L. Seip, C.M. Maresh, W.J. Kraemer, J.S. Volek, Dietary carbohydrate restriction improves insulin sensitivity, blood pressure, microvascular function, and cellular adhesion markers in individuals taking statins, Nutr. Res. 33(11) (2013) 905-12.

[28] E.A. Argao, J.E. Heubi, Fat-soluble vitamin deficiency in infants and children, Curr. Opin. Pediatr. 5(5) (1993) 562-6.

[29] Q.Y. Eng, P.V. Thanikachalam, S. Ramamurthy, Molecular understanding of Epigallocatechin gallate (EGCG) in cardiovascular and metabolic diseases, J. Ethnopharmacol. 210 (2018) 296-310.

[30] R.A. Wilson, W. Deasy, C.G. Stathis, A. Hayes, M.B. Cooke, Intermittent Fasting with or without Exercise Prevents Weight Gain and Improves Lipids in Diet-Induced Obese Mice, Nutrients 10(3) (2018).

[31] E. Dybkowska, A. Sadowska, F. Swiderski, R. Rakowska, K. Wysocka, The occurrence of

resveratrol in foodstuffs and its potential for supporting cancer prevention and treatment. A review, Rocz. Panstw. Zakl. Hig. 69(1) (2018) 5-14.

[32] P.R. Gibson, S.J. Shepherd, Evidence-based dietary management of functional gastrointestinal symptoms: The FODMAP approach, J. Gastroenterol. Hepatol. 25(2) (2010) 252-8.